T0324816

Duplicity Theory of Vision

The duplicity theory of vision concerns the comparisons (both differences and similarities) and interaction between the cone and rod systems in the visual pathways, with the assumption that the cone system is active during daylight vision and the rod system functions in low light (night vision). Research on this aspect of vision dates back to the seventeenth century and the work of Newton, and is still ongoing today. This book describes the origin and development of this fundamental theory within vision research – whilst also examining the Young-Helmholtz trichromatic colour theory, and the opponent colour theory of Hering – and presents evidence and ideas in the light of modern conceptions of the theory. Written for academic researchers and graduate students, the book reviews knowledge of the tradition of duplicity theory, inspiring questions related to anatomy, comparative biology, molecular biology, photochemistry, physiology, genetics, phylogenetics and psychophysics.

BJØRN AND ULF STABELL have worked in close collaboration on vision research at the Institute of Psychology, University of Oslo, since 1964. For 45 years their research has focussed on questions related to the duplicity theory of vision, publishing over 70 papers. Since 1986, the Stabells have been recipients of State Scholarships of Norway. During the first years of their studies they used a Hecht and Schlaer adaptometer (the 1938 version), being inspired by the papers of P. Saugstad and A. Saugstad (1959) and I. Lie (1963). In 1970 a copy of W. D. Wright's colorimeter at Imperial College of Science, London, became available at the institute (built by B. Hisdal). Now W. D. Wright's and J. D. Moreland's well-known papers became the main focus of their interest. These authors had developed ingenious methods for investigating colour vision in the extrafoveal retina. By using the new Wright colorimeter and by modifying their methods somewhat, it was possible to obtain accurate data on sensitivity and colour vision functions from all regions of the retina, even from its most peripheral parts.

Duplicity Theory of Vision

From Newton to the Present

Edited by

BJØRN STABELL AND ULF STABELL

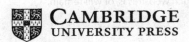

CAMBRIDGE
UNIVERSITY PRESS

University Printing House, Cambridge CB2 8BS, United Kingdom

Cambridge University Press is part of the University of Cambridge.

It furthers the University's mission by disseminating knowledge in the pursuit of education, learning and research at the highest international levels of excellence.

www.cambridge.org
Information on this title: www.cambridge.org/9780521111171

© B. Stabell and U. Stabell 2009

First published 2009

A catalogue record for this publication is available from the British Library

Library of Congress Cataloguing in Publication data
Stabell, Bjørn.
  The duplicity theory of vision : from Newton to the present / Bjørn Stabell,
  Ulf Stabell.
     p.   cm.
  Includes bibliographical references and index.
  ISBN 978-0-521-11117-1 (hardback)
  1. Visual pathways.   2. Eye–Adaptation.   3. Vision–Research–History.
  I. Stabell, Ulf.   II. Title.
  QP475.S685 2009
  612.8´4–dc22   2009022355

ISBN 978-0-521-11117-1 Hardback

Additional resources for this publication at :
www.cambridge.org/9780521111171

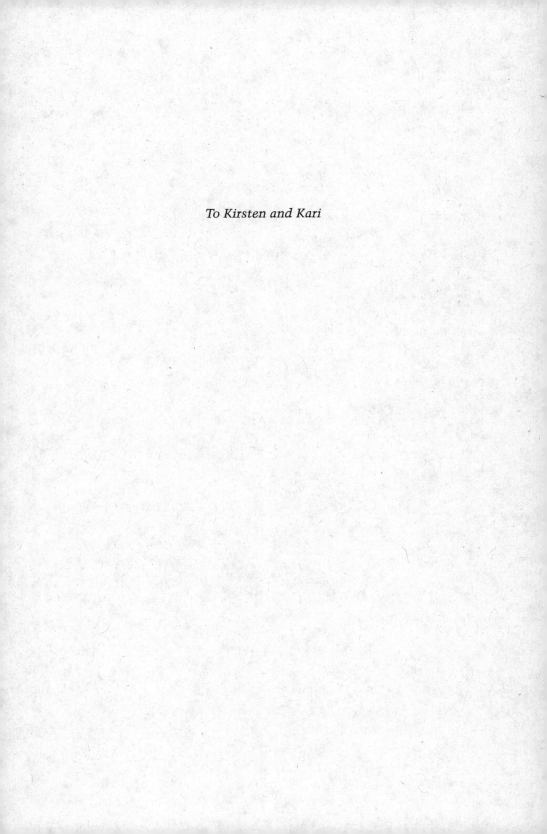

To Kirsten and Kari

Contents

Acknowledgements

We gratefully acknowledge the expert guidance during the whole publication process by the editors and publication staff of Cambridge University Press: Martin Griffiths (Commissioning Editor, Neuroscience & Animal Behaviour), Stacey Meade (Publishing Assistant), Alison C. Evans (Assistant Editor, Life Sciences), and Jonathan Ratcliffe (Production Editor). Furthermore, we want to thank Judith Shaw (freelance copy-editor for Cambridge University Press), who presented many relevant queries, offered valuable advice and constructive criticism, and copy-edited the typescript of the book. Lastly, we want to thank Kirsten E. Stabell for her help in solving many intricate linguistic problems and for excellent and faithful secretarial assistance during the publication process.

1 **Introduction**

1.1 ROOTS OF THE DUPLICITY THEORY OF VISION: ANCIENT GREEKS

The duplicity theory is the most basic and comprehensive theory within vision research. Yet, there has been no attempt to describe its developmental history. In the present work, therefore, our aim has been to throw some light on this dark area in the history of science. As will be seen, the duplicity theory is not an old, static, antiquated theory dating back to Schultze's (1866) original formulation of the theory, as is generally held, but is a living body that expands and deepens as new knowledge of the rod and cone systems is obtained.

The beginning of the scientific study of vision may be traced back to the Ancient Greeks. However, due to an almost complete lack of knowledge about optics and sensory information processing at that time, the Greeks made two serious mistakes in their functional interpretation of the visual system. Thus, they generally held that (1) the crystalline lens of the eye was the most important organ of vision, being the actual sense organ, and (2) visual perception depended in a fundamental way on some sort of 'rays' that emanated *from* the lens *toward* the objects of the environment.

Both assumptions were accepted and adhered to in one form or other by many of the leading Ancient Greek philosophers and research workers. The most important among them, because of his strong and long-lasting influence on science in Western Europe, was Galen – also named Galenos (about AD 130–200). He presumed that visual perception depended on a 'pneuma' or 'visual spirit' that originated in the brain and circulated through the hollow optic nerve filling the crystalline lens in the eye. Thereby, it could confer the ability of perception to the lens.

The question of how the lens acquired information about the environment was answered, in accord with the generally held 'lantern' or 'emission' theory, by the assumption that the lens emitted some sort of 'rays' in the form of a cone that touched objects in the outer world. (The common observation that the eyes of animals may appear luminous like lanterns when seen in night vision supported the theory.)

The remaining question of how individuals obtained information about the environment from these 'rays' could be answered in accord with the 'likeness' principle. This principle presupposed that each object in the world could be characterized by a particular composition of the four basic elements ('earth', 'water', 'air' and 'fire'), which the Ancient Greeks believed formed the substance of the world, and that the 'water' element of the emitted outgoing 'rays' could gain knowledge about the 'water' elements of objects, the 'earth' element knowledge about the 'earth' elements, and so on, giving the individual complete knowledge of the perceived objects.

However, not all leading authorities accepted this generally held information theory. Aristotle (384–322 BC), for instance, rejected the 'lantern' theory on the well-known fact that humans do not see anything in complete darkness. In contrast to the 'lantern' theory he considered light to be an activity or a movement of an ether-like substance originating in luminous or illuminated bodies and transmitted through the transparent media of the environment to the eyes.

Democritus (460–370 BC) also rejected the 'lantern' theory and suggested that light consisted of particles that were transmitted *from* the objects *towards* the eye. More important, he advanced the seminal suggestion that the *perception* of an object and the 'real' object may differ considerably, since both the environment between the object and the body, and the sense organ itself, may change the messenger particles significantly. Colour, for instance, was not considered as part of 'real' objects, which he thought were composed of 'atoms'.

Such hypotheses and theories that deviated from the mainstream were, however, largely ignored or treated with ridicule until as late as the seventeenth century, when Kepler, Huygens, Hooke and Newton entered the stage. The two serious errors had then been dominating thinking for about two millennia (see Polyak (1948) for an excellent review of the ancient conception of the structure and function of the visual organ, and also Goethe's (1810) historical review).

Nevertheless, the Ancient Greeks, although led far astray in their thinking about visual information processing, may be seen as the originators of the scientific study of vision. Indeed, even the roots of the duplicity theory may be found in their research. Thus, the Ancient Greeks discovered that the ability to see by day and night differs markedly between animal species. Empedocles (fifth century BC) attempted to explain this difference by suggesting that it was due to differences in the relative amount of 'fire' and 'water' in the inner eye. A relatively small amount of 'fire' or 'water' produced poor night and day vision, respectively (Goethe, 1810, pp. 524–525, and p. 530). Similarly, Theophrastus (the successor of Aristotle at the Lyceum at Athens) suggested that nocturnal animals may see much better than humans by night due to more of the 'fire' element in their eyes. Interestingly, he also suggested that 'fire' from the sun may drastically reduce the amount of 'fire' in the eye and, thereby, reduce the ability to see by night (Hanssen, 2000).

1.2 FURTHER DEVELOPMENT OF THE DUPLICITY THEORY

Further progress in our understanding of the differences in visual processing in day and night vision had to wait for about 2000 years. Thus, the first modern breakthrough was accomplished by Schultze (1866). Based on comparative histological as well as psychophysical evidence, he suggested that (1) night and day vision were mediated, respectively, by rod and cone receptors in the retina, (2) the cones mediated both achromatic and chromatic sensations, while the rods mediated achromatic vision only, (3) the rod and cone systems functioned independently of each other, and (4) the cones provided for better spatial resolution. (For an evaluation of Schultze's duplicity theory, see Saugstad & Saugstad (1959).)

The theory that the human retina contains two basically different types of photoreceptor (rods and cones) that function independently of each other and operate under different conditions, giving rise to qualitatively different colour sensations, brought about a paradigm shift within vision research. Thus, the theory eventually became generally accepted and introduced a fundamentally new understanding of visual functioning. Schultze's theory also generated new fundamental questions with regards to differences and similarities as well as possible interactions between the information processing of the two receptor systems.

Obviously, answers to these questions presuppose knowledge of the characteristics of both the rod and cone mechanisms. Knowledge about basic characteristics of cones had long been accumulated within the Newton-Young-Maxwell-Helmholtz tradition (in the following referred to as the 'Newton tradition'), but little was known about rod functioning at the time Schultze (1866) published his important paper. The ignorance of the functioning of the rod receptor system is clearly revealed in Helmholtz's 'Handbuch' (1867, p. 214). Actually, at this developmental stage of research, he could find no conclusive evidence of *any* rod contribution to vision. No wonder, then, that the theory of Schultze did not gain immediate general acceptance.

In the following years, however, knowledge about basic rod functions developed rapidly within the Schultze-Boll-Kühne-Parinaud-König tradition (in the following termed the 'Schultze tradition') and strong evidence supporting and extending Schultze's theory emerged.

Early in the twentieth century, then, his theory had become generally accepted. Von Kries, a leading authority on vision, was its strongest defender and also coined the term 'Duplizitätstheorie' (duplicity theory; see von Kries, 1929). Perhaps his most important contribution, though, was his attempt to integrate the evidence accumulated within the Newton and Schultze traditions into a more comprehensive duplicity theory (von Kries, 1911).

Yet, the development of the duplicity theory was also profoundly influenced by a third research tradition (in the following termed the

'Goethe tradition') that started with Goethe, who believed that the phenomenological analysis of colour sensation in its own right would reveal the basic laws of colour vision (see Goethe, 1810). A great step forward within this tradition was taken when Hering pointed out that the phenomenological character of colour vision may also provide information with regard to the material processes underlying the phenomenological experiences. Indeed, on the basis of his phenomenological analysis of colour vision, Hering – in opposition to Newton, Helmholtz and Schultze – could conclude that the basic physiological colour-related processes had to *interact* and *oppose* each other somewhere in the visual pathway (see Hering, 1878).

Surprisingly, von Kries made no serious attempt to integrate the evidence provided by this third tradition into his theory. Thus, it was left to G. E. Müller (1896, 1897, 1923, 1930), who was deeply rooted in the Goethe tradition, to develop a duplicity theory that incorporated the evidence procured within all these three major research traditions.

Hence, the theory of G. E. Müller may be seen to represent the end of the first phase of the development of the duplicity theory. In order to review this first phase, we will describe the contribution of each of the three different research traditions and we start with the Newton tradition.

Part I   The development of the basic ideas of the duplicity theory from Newton to G. E. Müller

2 The Newton tradition

2.1 NEWTON'S UNIVERSAL COLOUR THEORY

One major root of the duplicity theory as formulated by Schultze, von Kries and G. E. Müller is represented by the Newton tradition. Within this line of research a rudimentary understanding of the cone mechanisms developed, ending up with the formulation of the famous Young-Helmholtz trichromatic colour theory (Helmholtz, 1867). This theory profoundly influenced Schultze, von Kries and G. E. Müller in their attempt to construct their theories. In fact, the theory forms an integrated part of the duplicity theory and its development may therefore be seen to represent the starting point of the development of the duplicity theory.

Certainly, the development of the trichromatic theory was in many ways initiated by Newton's ingenious experiments and theories on light and colour. In fact, his contribution deserves to be ranked as *the first major paradigm shift within vision research in modern times*. Surprisingly, however, Newton's revolutionary ideas about light and colour are, today, not generally well known. In the following, therefore, we present his theories in some detail.

Newton's theories were first published 19 February 1672 as a letter in *Philosophical Transactions of the Royal Society of London* (1671/1672). His most important ideas about light and colour are stated below in his own words. They are given in his propositions 1, 2, 3, 7 and 13 (see also Cohen, 1978, pp. 53–57).

> 1. As the Rays of light differ in degrees of Refrangibility, so they also differ in their disposition to exhibit this or that particular colour. Colours are not *Qualifications of Light*, derived from Refractions,

or Reflections of natural Bodies (as 'tis generally believed,) but *Original and connate properties*, which in divers Rays are divers.

2. To the same degree of Refrangibility ever belongs the same colour, and to the same colour ever belongs the same degree of Refrangibility.

3. The species of colour, and degree of Refrangibility proper to any particular sort of Rays, is not mutable by Refraction, nor by Reflection from natural bodies, nor by any other cause, that I could yet observe.

7. But the most surprising, and wonderful composition was that of *Whiteness*. There is no one sort of Rays which alone can exhibit this. 'Tis ever compounded, and to its composition are requisite all the aforesaid primary Colours, mixed in a due proportion.

13. ... the Colours of all natural Bodies have no other origin than this, that they are variously qualified to reflect one sort of light in greater plenty then another.

Later, on the basis of very extensive experimental research, Newton formulated his universal colour theory, where he suggested that all colours in the universe, which are generated by light, are colours of either homogenous or compounded lights and that, when quantities and types of rays that excite the eye are given, then the colour of the light is known (Newton, 1730, pp.154–161). In his own words,

> And therefore if the reason of any Colour whatever be required, we have nothing else to do than to consider how the Rays in the Sun's Light have by Reflexions and Refractions, or other causes, been parted from one another, or mixed together; or otherwise to find out what sorts of Rays are in the Light by which that Colour is made, and in what Proportion (Newton, 1730, p. 160).

2.2 AN ALTERNATIVE TO NEWTON'S THEORIES OF LIGHT AND COLOUR

Newton's (1671/1672) paper represents one of the most important contributions in the history of science. In order to adequately appreciate this eminent contribution, it is necessary to pay due attention to the generally held view with regard to light and colour at the time the paper was published. Thus, the originality of Newton's paper is best apprehended by comparing his theories on light and colour with contemporary theories (Cohen, 1978, pp. 208–209). An illustrative example of the contemporary viewpoints is given by the colour theory of Hooke, a brilliant scientist on whom the Royal Society of London relied to evaluate Newton's paper (Cohen, 1978, pp. 110–115).

Despite the fact that Newton's discourse had been received with much applause at the Society's meeting, Hooke's referee report, delivered only a few days later, comparing the explanatory value of Newton's and his own colour theory, was severely critical. Hooke argued that his own colour theory could explain more simply not only his own experimental results but also those presented by Newton, and that it was useless in scientific theory construction to multiply entities without necessity in the way Newton had done. Thus, opposed to the basic assumption of Newton that 'white' sensation was linked to a complex physical stimulus, the available evidence seemed to Hooke to prove that 'white' light was nothing but primitive, simple, uniform and transverse pulses or waves propagated through a homogeneous, uniform and transparent medium (the ether). Whiteness and blackness were accordingly assumed to represent nothing but large and small quantities of this light. Chromatic, prismatic colours, on the other hand, were explained by the assumption that the uniform, simple motion of white light became blended or mixed with adventitious motions when it fell obliquely on a refracting medium. The part of the light refracted least was assumed to give the impression of red, the part refracted most blue, while all the intermediate colours in the spectrum were thought to be determined by intermixing of the red and blue light. Hence, all chromatic colours in the world, except red and blue, were assumed to be caused by compound pulses made of the red and blue primary pulses only. Finally, Hooke assumed that the adventitious motions could be destroyed by other motions when compounded lights were united anew. The original, simple white light could thereby be restored.

Today, it is of interest to note that Newton's more complex theory prevailed. Thus, Newton's most conspicuous and original hypotheses, that the light stimulus that generated the apparently simple sensation of white was compounded and determined by primary lights mixed in due proportion, and that the solar spectrum consisted of an innumerable number of different lights linked to different hue sensations, were later embraced by Young, Maxwell and Helmholtz.

On the other hand, faced with Thomas Young's famous double slit experiment, where he explained the interference pattern obtained by the wave concept of light, and the test experiment carried out by François Aragon in 1819, that came out strongly in favour of the wave model of Augustin Fresnel, the scientific community in the early 1800s abandoned Newton's corpuscular theory of light in favour of the wave theory (see Gribbin, 2003, pp. 403–410).

Newton knew that there had to be an intimate relation between light and waves, but did not consider the wave aspect to be an intrinsic part of his concept of light. Thus, he wrote, 'For, assuming the rays of light to be small bodies emitted every way from shining substances, those, when they impinge on any refracting or reflecting superficies, must as necessarily excite vibration in the æther, as stones do in water when thrown into it' (see Newton, 1675, p. 179, 193–194).

It should be noted, however, that Newton's corpuscular theory of light gained renewed interest in 1905, when Einstein explained the photoelectric effect by Planck's quantum principle and so was led to postulate the existence of 'quanta' of light.

At present, it is generally held that photons have both particle- and wave-like attributes. (For modern notions about elementary and force particles including the photon, see Greene, 2005, pp. 84–95, 180–199, 344–360.)

It is of interest to note that a controversy concerning the nature of light similar to that between Newton and Hooke took place between Democritus and Aristotle. While Democritus held that objects could be seen through an empty space, Aristotle assumed that movement of a medium between the objects and the eye was necessary for seeing the objects. In fact, Aristotle assumed that movement of a medium was also a necessary condition for the sensation of sound, smell, touch and taste (see Goethe, 1810, p. 533–534).

2.3 PHOTOTRANSDUCTION IN THE RETINA AND SIGNAL TRANSMISSION TO THE BRAIN: NEWTON'S SPECULATIONS

In his attempt to explain the strict connection between rays and colour, Newton (1675), in his second paper on light and colour, suggested that the rays excited vibration in an ethereal medium when they impinged upon the ends of the capilamenta of the optic nerve in the retina. Depending on the size and strength of the rays, they were thought to excite vibrations of various sizes. As the rays became bigger and stronger, the vibrations became larger. These vibrations, then, were thought to run through the optic nerve (as the corpuscles themselves could not do) to the sensorium and there affect the sense with various colours according to their size and mixture. The largest vibrations produced red, the middle green, and the smallest violet, while white could be generated by mixing all the different vibrations in due proportion. No interaction between the ethereal waves and no change in quality occurred in the optic nerve. Thus, the different qualities of colour seen were assumed to depend on the interpretation made by the sensorium.

Interestingly, Newton hypothesized that the vibrations of the retina and the eardrum were conveyed to the sensorium by similar processes. In fact, he speculated that *all* types of sensation were transmitted by vibration of the ethereal medium (see Newton, 1730, p. 353). Thus, it appears that Newton anticipated Johannes Müller's famous 'specific nerve-energy' doctrine by more than 100 years. Indeed, he correctly attributed the different types of sensory quality to the brain, and not to activities of nerves leading to the brain, as Johannes Müller's doctrine most often has been read. It seems fair to add, however, that Johannes Müller did not take a firm stand on whether the essential cause of the different qualities was to be found in the nerves themselves or in the brain (see Müller, 1840, p. 261).

2.4 NEWTON'S GRAVITATION PRINCIPLE APPLIED TO COLOUR MIXTURE DATA

A third major contribution by Newton is represented by his ideas of colour mixture. These ingenious ideas paved the way for Maxwell's fundamental discovery of the triplicity of colour vision, that is, that colour vision depended on three types of receptor at the retinal level (Maxwell, 1855, 1860).

Thus, in order to illustrate the results of colour mixture, Newton represented the colours of the spectrum on the circumference of a circle, making the colours gradually pass into one another as they do when generated by a prism (see Newton, 1730, pp. 154–158). Although Newton held that there existed a very large number of different colour sensations, he assumed that the number of primary colours was restricted to seven (red, orange, yellow, green, blue, indigo and violet). These seven primary colours were represented on the circumference of the colour circle by dividing it into seven parts proportional to the seven musical string intervals that establish an octave as illustrated in Fig. 2.1. Taking advantage of his principle of gravitation, he could then present the colour mixture laws graphically in a two-dimensional colour space. Thus, in the middle of each of the seven arcs he placed a small circle, the centre of which represented the centre of gravity of the rays of the corresponding primary colour, and the number of rays of the colour, the gravitational force. The common centre of gravity of all the primary colours in the mixture, then, represented the location of the resultant colour. When the common centre of gravity was located on the circumference of the circle, the colour would appear saturated to the highest degree, while it would gradually appear more whitish and eventually become white as its location approached the centre of the circle.

These ideas of colour mixture make Newton the principal forerunner of modern colorimetry. Thus, it can be seen that both

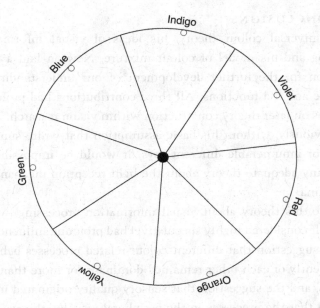

Fig. 2.1 The colour circle of Newton representing the visual spectrum. Although Newton held that the prismatic spectrum consisted of innumerable different sorts of rays, he assumed that the number of primary colours was restricted to seven.

the centre of gravity principle of colour mixture (implying additivity of colour matches) and the concept of spectral composition of light stimuli were clearly spelled out by Newton.

Not all colour-mixture data, however, could readily be handled by Newton's model. He found that when two colours opposite to each other in the colour circle were mixed in due proportions, so that the common centre of gravity fell on the centre of the circle, the colour mixture did not generate a perfect white. Mixing four or five (or possibly three) primary colours, however, was sufficient. A further complication was observed when primary red and violet were mixed. In such instances he found the resultant colour to be purple, which was not a prismatic colour and, therefore, did not fit well with his model of colour mixture. (See Helmholtz, 1855, for a discussion.)

2.5 CONCLUSIONS

By his universal colour theory, his ideas of visual information processing and his model of colour mixture, Newton laid a solid foundation for the further development of our understanding of both cone and rod functions. All three contributions had profound influences on later theory construction within vision research.

Obviously, without his basic assumption that white sunlight consists of innumerable different rays, it would be impossible to develop any adequate theory about the light reception mechanisms in the retina.

Also, his theory about visual information processing (which he himself considered highly speculative) had profound influence. In fact, the suggestion that different colour-related processes behaved independently of each other remained dominant for more than two centuries, and the suggestion that sensory quality originated in the brain and that the processes in the peripheral visual pathways only differed quantitatively are still generally accepted.

The third major contribution (his ingenious model of colour mixture, where he applied his principle of gravitation to describe the colour-mixture data) paved the way for Maxwell's discovery of the triplicity of colour vision. It also allowed the prediction that the primary colour-related processes would behave independently of each other in the light reception process. It is important to note, however, that the colour-mixture data obtained did not prove Newton's assumption that different colour-related processes remained independent of each other during the whole journey from retina to brain as several vision research workers later mistakenly believed (see Wright, 1946, pp 146–152).

2.6 YOUNG'S COLOUR THEORY: THREE INSTEAD OF SEVEN PRIMARIES

Newton did not present any strong argument in support of his assumption of seven primary colours and it was challenged by the well-known fact that painters could produce any object colour by mixing only three pigment colours: red, yellow and blue, called the three primaries (green was in general assumed to represent a secondary colour, since it could be produced by mixing blue and yellow). There have been many attempts to explain this apparent triplicity of colour vision. Weale (1957) has given an interesting account of trichromatic ideas in the seventeenth and eighteenth centuries. He emphasizes the theories of Lomonosow and Palmer, proposed in 1756 and 1777, respectively. They both suggested that there were three different types of light and three different types of retinal molecule. Each type of retinal molecule was thought to be activated by its analogous type of ray, giving rise to red, yellow and blue sensations

Given the enormous authority of Newton and his convincing experiments, it appears surprising that both Lomonosow and Palmer opposed his basic assumption that white light from the sun is a mixture of innumerable kinds of different rays that are linked to different hue sensations (see Newton, 1671/1672, props. 1, 2 and 7). The acceptance of Newton's assumption leads to a quite different explanation of the triplicity of colour vision. Thus, it would follow that the essential cause of the apparent triplicity should be sought for solely in the visual system. This lead was followed by Young (1802a), who was well acquainted with Newton's ideas. He suggested that there existed three different kinds of particle or resonator in the retina which were maximally sensitive to different wavelengths. The activity of the different resonators was assumed to be independently conveyed to the sensorium and there give rise to three different kinds of colour sensations. At first, he assumed that the three primary activities gave rise to red, yellow and blue in the brain (Young, 1802a), but later he chose red, green and violet colours as primaries (Young, 1802b, 1807).

Yet, as pointed out by Helmholtz (1852), the finding by artists that all object colours may be reproduced by mixing red, yellow and blue pigments could not be a basis for colour theory construction, since the composition of the spectral lights reflected from pigments could not be adequately controlled. Thus, as already explained by

Newton (1730, pp.179–185, 245–288), a pigment may absorb, transmit and reflect the spectral lights that fall upon it and when two pigments are mixed, the new compound pigment reflects and transmits only those rays that are not absorbed by each of the two pigments. This complexity, of course, prevented an adequate control of the spectral composition of the light that entered the subject's eye. Moreover, both Newton (1730, pp.132–134) and Helmholtz (1852) stressed that the experimenter could not control the composition of the spectral lights by the apparent colour of the pigment either, since the same colour sensation could be a composite of different spectral lights (the metamerism of colours).

On the other hand, when monochromatic *prismatic* lights were mixed and focused on the retina, the different rays that entered the eye were combined additively and could easily be controlled and varied by the experimenter. Thus, as was first clearly explained by Newton (1730) and later by Helmholtz (1852), mixing of pigments and mixing of spectral lights generated a subtractive and an additive result, respectively.

Another serious problem confronting the trichromatic colour theory of Young (1807) was the observation of Helmholtz (1852) that monochromatic spectral colours could *not* be reproduced by mixing three primary spectral lights. Thus, he found that prismatic yellow and blue colours could not be matched by mixing, respectively, red and green, and green and violet lights. The spectral colours were found to be more saturated than the mixtures. Adding another primary to the mixture would only enhance the saturation differences found. Helmholtz (1852) concluded that there had to be at least five so-called primary colours.

2.7 MAXWELL: TRIPLICITY OF COLOUR VISION PROVED

The results of Maxwell's (1855, 1860) colour matching experiments, however, showed this conclusion to be wrong and the trichromatic colour theory of Young to be on the right lines. Maxwell's treatment of his experimental results was based on Newton's ideas of colour mixture. Thus, he presumed that the method of determining the position and strength of the resultant colour of mixed lights is mathematically identical to that of finding the centre of gravity of weights and placing a weight equal to the sum of the weights at the point so found. This presumption presupposes that colour mixing is additive. If, for example, the same light is added to or subtracted from both test and comparison fields, which have been matched with respect to all colour aspects, it is assumed that the match will still hold; or if two matched lights (A and B) are added to two other matched lights (C and D), the result is two lights that match, that is, (A+C) match (B+D). As Helmholtz (1855, p. 24) puts it, 'Gleich aussehende Farben gemischt geben gleich aussehende Mischungen' (mixing equally appearing colours gives equally appearing mixtures). Hence, Maxwell (taking account of Newton's laws of gravitation) could express his colour-mixture results *algebraically* in the form of equations with the colour under test on one side of the equation and the mixture of three standard lights (red, green and blue) on the other.

Thus, Maxwell (1860) first made a colour match between a mixture of his standard red, green and blue lights and a constant reference white. He then replaced one of the standard primaries by the monochromatic spectral light to be studied, and a new match of the constant white was made. Now he had two equations for the match of the same standard white and could subtract one from the other to obtain the equation of the unknown spectral light investigated. By this procedure, Maxwell (1860) discovered that the colour effects of all monochromatic spectral lights could, in fact, be matched by using only three primaries. Hence, he had proved that the retinal colour response to spectral lights must involve a triplex mechanism. Since there was no histological evidence for such a triplex mechanism at the time, the triple subdivision had to occur on a sub-microscopic scale.

His mathematical treatment was as follows:

Given that the three standard lights are denoted R, G and B, white sensation W, the spectral light to be studied S and a, b, c,

d and e are measurements of normalized light intensity, then the chromaticity of the unknown spectral light $f(S)$ may be calculated. Thus when for instance:

$a(R) + b(G) + c(B) = W = d(R) + e(G) + f(S)$, then

$a(R) + b(G) + c(B) = d(R) + e(G) + f(S)$ and

$f(S) = (a - d)(R) + (b - e)(G) + c(B)$

(It should be noted that the equals sign, '=', reads; 'is matched by'.)

As will be seen, the application of Newton's law of gravity made allowance for an algebraic treatment of the colour-mixture data and, hence, for the use of negative values of standard lights. The problem pointed out by Helmholtz (1852), that monochromatic spectral lights are too saturated to be matched by a mixture of primaries, could then be resolved on the assumption that each of the three receptors is activated by a large part of the spectrum. The mixture of two or three primaries may, therefore, activate the white component mechanism more than monochromatic spectral lights and, hence, be less saturated. In accord with this assumption, Maxwell (1860) showed that by adding one of the three standard lights to the spectral test light it could be desaturated (i.e. the white component of the spectral test light could be increased) to such an extent that it could be matched by the mixture of the two other standard lights.

The evidence provided by Maxwell (1855, 1860) was generally taken as conclusive evidence in favour of the basic assumption that the central fovea contains three different types of receptor. Thus, it was argued that if colours were determined by the relative activity of three independent receptor processes in the retina, then, by the use of three standard stimuli, one should be capable of stimulating the receptor systems in all possible combinations and, thereby, reproducing any of the spectral colours as demonstrated by Maxwell (1855, 1860).

Maxwell adduced further strong evidence in favour of the triplicity of the normal retina by demonstrating that a protanope ('red'-colour-blind) could match every colour in the spectrum by using only two primaries. In fact, his results suggested that the protanope

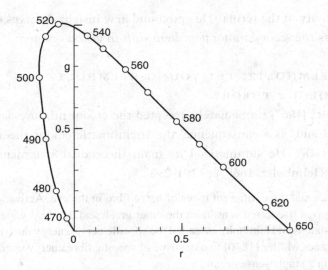

Fig. 2.2 Chromaticity coordinates of monochromatic spectral lights measured at the central fovea in a dark-adapted state and expressed in the WDW (i.e. W. D. Wright) diagram. Thus, the data points are plotted in terms of the matching stimuli 650, 530 and 460 nm and the normalized units are based on matches of 582.5 and 494 nm. That is, the amount of the 650 nm and 530 nm stimuli required to match 582.5 nm were regarded as equal, as were the amounts of 530 nm and 460 nm stimuli required to match 494 nm.

had a reduced form of colour vision in that the red mechanism was lacking (Maxwell, 1855, 1860, 1872).

On the basis of his discovery that all spectral lights can be matched by using only three standard lights, and by using Grassmann's (1853) vector diagram for representation of resultant colours, Maxwell (1860) could present his colour matching results graphically in a two-dimensional colour space by an equilateral triangle (the Maxwell colour triangle). (Fig. 2.2 gives an example of a modern representation of colours of monochromatic spectral lights in a two-dimensional colour space.)

The conclusions of Maxwell (1855, 1860) departed from the colour theory of Newton in two important respects: (1) He made use of only three primaries, and (2) he found the essential cause of the triplicity in the retina. This profound new insight deserves to be ranked as *the second major paradigm shift in vision research.*

2.8 HELMHOLTZ: THE YOUNG-HELMHOLTZ COLOUR THEORY

Helmholtz (1867) immediately accepted the colour-mixture data of Maxwell and, as a consequence, the trichromatic colour theory of Young (1807). He summarized its main theoretical statements as follows (Helmholtz, 1867, pp. 291–292):

1. There exist three different types of nerve fibre in the eye. Activation of one gives rise to red sensation, the other green and the third violet. (In this statement Helmholtz extended the specific nerve-energy doctrine of Johannes Müller (1840) to a doctrine of specific fibre energy operating within a single sense organ.)
2. The three types of fibre are activated to different degrees by different wavelengths in that red-related fibres are most strongly activated by the longest wavelengths, the green-related fibres by middle wavelengths, while the violet-related fibres are most strongly activated by the shortest wavelengths.
3. Pure yellow results from moderate activity in red- and green-related fibres and a small activation of violet-related fibres, while blue is produced by moderate activities of green- and violet-related fibres and a small activation of red-related fibres. Finally, white sensation is produced when the three different typses of nerve fibre are activated to about the same degree.
4. The nerve activities of the three different types of fibre are qualitatively different and transmitted to the brain without interacting with each other.

As an alternative possibility, Helmholtz (1867, p. 292) pointed out that the triplex mechanism might be based on three independent and qualitatively different processes *within each fibre.* Under this alternative, an essential cause of the triplicity and colour quality would be seated in each nerve fibre.

Later, in the 1896 edition of his 'Handbuch', however, he, in accord with Newton (1675, 1730), attributed the different types of sensory quality solely to the brain. Here he assumed that there were no qualitative differences as regards nerve conduction, so that the nerve fibres were like telegraph wires which passively conduct electricity.

Of course, Helmholtz knew that the ether waves of light did not directly activate the nerve fibres. Instead, he assumed that the nerve activity was generated by processes in light-sensitive elements, and that these elements had to be cones, since only cones were found in the central fovea, where vision was best developed, and also because vision deteriorated with eccentricity, where the number of rods relative to cones increased. The transformation of light to nerve impulses (the phototransduction in the receptors) was, however, completely unknown in the 1860s (Helmholtz, 1867, pp. 214–215).

3 The Schultze tradition

3.1 THE DUPLICITY THEORY OF MAX SCHULTZE

The first section of Helmholtz's classical 'Handbuch der Physiologischen Optik' was published in 1856, the second (containing the Young-Helmholtz trichromatic colour theory) in 1860, the third partly at the beginning and partly towards the close of 1866, while the complete work was published in 1867. The Young-Helmholtz colour theory was, therefore, known to Max Schultze (professor in anatomy and the director of the Anatomic Institute in Bonn, Germany) when he published his important work in 1866. Indeed, he accepted its major assumption that three different cone fibres conveyed independent, qualitatively different colour-related processes.

Yet, in addition to the cone receptors and their functions, he introduced the much more numerous rod receptors presuming that they were responsible for night vision, and that they mediated achromatic sensation only. This theory of Schultze may be seen as *the third major paradigm shift in vision research*. It entailed a profound new insight into visual processing and generated basic questions about differences and similarities as well as about possible interactions between the information processing of the two different receptor systems.

3.2 EVIDENCE IN FAVOUR OF THE THEORY

Schultze's hypothesis that the retina contained two basically different kinds of receptor was based on extensive, comparative histological studies. Although he was aware of the fact that the structure of a receptor type in different species, and even in the same retina, may differ markedly, he found rods and cones *in general* to differ both with respect to structure and occurrence. Thus, he pointed to several characteristics that may be summarized as follows (Schultze, 1866, pp. 247–251):

1. Rods are generally longer than cones, and the rod and cone outer segments have rod- and cone-like shapes, respectively, as the names indicate.
2. The terminal of the inner segment of the cones is much thicker than that of the rods and divides into several thin fibres.
3. Cones of many diurnal bird species possess yellow, red or colourless strongly light-refracting droplets (globules) between their inner and outer segments, positioned so that light has to pass through them before reaching the outer segment.
4. Several diurnal (lizard, snake, etc.) and nocturnal (bat, mole, shark, hedgehog, mouse, skate, etc.) species have only cone and rod retinas, respectively.
5. The central fovea of humans, apes and falcons contains only cones.

Based on points 4 and 5, Schultze (1866) concluded that cones and rods mediated day and night vision, respectively, and that both receptor systems functioned as light and space receptors. In order to decide whether both receptor systems might also mediate chromatic sensation, Schultze (1866) compared day and night vision in humans. He referred to the extensive study of Aubert (1865) who had found that colour vision changed qualitatively during dark adaptation with a gradual transition from chromatic to achromatic vision where, eventually, only brightness differences were observed. Consequently, Schultze (1866) concluded that only the cone receptor system could mediate chromatic vision. In accordance with this conclusion, he pointed to the fact that colour vision deteriorated when a test field was moved outward from the rod-free fovea, while the number of rod receptors activated increased.

3.3 ONE OR SEVERAL TYPES OF CONE?

Having presented strong arguments in favour of the assumption that only cones may mediate chromatic colour vision, Schultze (1866) sought to develop his theory a step further by attempting to answer the fundamental question of whether there were one or several types of cone in the retina.

In his investigation of the retinas of mammals and fish he could find no anatomical evidence for different types of cone representing the three different primaries of the Young-Helmholtz colour theory – the cones appeared essentially similar. Hence, he had to conclude that these retinas contained only one type of cone. Yet, he could point to another characteristic of the cones that might account for the triplicity of colour vision: each cone had several outgoing fibres connected to the inner segment, while the rod receptors had only one fibre connected. Reasoning from the plausible assumption that each cone needed several fibres in order to handle both achromatic and chromatic information processing, while a rod receptor, mediating a simple achromatic sensation, needed only one fibre, he came to the conclusion that the different fibres connected to each cone receptor were capable of reacting in a qualitatively different manner when excited by light of different colours (Schultze, 1866, p. 258). Thus, Schultze, in effect, suggested that the different fibres connected to the inner segment of each cone in mammalian and fish retinas constituted the basis for colour vision, serving independent, qualitatively different nerve processes.

In the retinas of diurnal birds, on the other hand, he *did* find evidence for three different kinds of cone receptor. Thus, he found cones with red, yellow and colourless droplets (globules) situated at the junction of the inner and outer segments, so that light had to penetrate them before entering the outer segments. The droplets, therefore, appeared to function as colour filters, and Schultze came to the conclusion that these different cone receptor types represented, respectively, the red, green and violet receptor mechanisms of the Young-Helmholtz colour theory. As an alternative, he suggested that cones with colourless droplets might function in a similar way to the cones of humans, being capable of generating the whole colour gamut.

The interesting finding that the outgoing fibre of the cones with coloured droplets was relatively thin and slender, like that of the rods, was interpreted as consistent with his prediction that each cone needed only one fibre when the retina contained several types of cone receptor.

Lastly, Schultze (1866) suggested that cones provided better spatial resolution than rods. However, presupposing that acuity was based on the number of receptors per unit retinal area, he encountered a serious problem when attempting to explain the reduction in acuity with retinal eccentricity. If each receptor sent an independent signal to the brain, acuity should increase, not deteriorate with eccentricity, due to the increasing number of small rods that far outnumbered the cones. In want of a better explanation of this apparent inconsistency, Schultze (1866) speculated that the better acuity performance of cones, somehow, was related to their ability to mediate colour vision. Thus, cones were assumed to perform better than rods in acuity tasks, because several fibres were connected to the inner segment of each cone and thereby provided greater information processing capability.

3.4 PHOTOTRANSDUCTION IS PHOTOCHEMICAL IN NATURE: BOLL AND KÜHNE

At the time Schultze (1866) published his duplicity theory, there was no consensus on phototransduction. Although it was known that light energy was transformed into nervous energy in the receptors, the transformation mechanism was completely unknown. Indeed, Newton's idea, presented nearly two centuries earlier, that light produced physical vibrations in the nerve fibres was still considered a viable alternative (Helmholtz, 1867, pp. 214–215).

The works of Boll and Kühne, published a few years later, however, were a breakthrough in our understanding of the phototransduction process. Boll (1877) discovered that the photopigment rhodopsin, situated in the outer segment of the rods, was bleached by light and regenerated in the dark and suggested that these photochemical processes might be a foundation of visual colour processing. Kühne (1879) disagreed with this suggestion and instead, on the basis of very extensive research, put forward his general 'optochemische Hypothese' (optochemical hypothesis) where he assumed the existence of photochemical see-substances (Sehstoff) both in rods and cones (Kühne, 1879, pp. 326–332).

This hypothesis may be said to supply a profound new insight and deserves to be ranked as *the fourth major paradigm shift within vision research*. Thus, based on the epoch-making contributions of Boll and Kühne, it soon became generally accepted that the phototransduction, in both rods and cones, was photochemical in nature.

3.5 BOLL: DISCOVERY OF RHODOPSIN AS A VISUAL PHOTOPIGMENT

As is sometimes the case, a great, new scientific discovery may be promoted by an unexpected observation brought about by accident. Franz Boll's marvellous discovery is an example. Thus, in Berlin in June 1876, he was to demonstrate the previously known red colour of the retina for the great Herman von Helmholtz among others. For this, he used frogs. He killed them by cutting off their heads. He then prepared the eyeball, bisected it with a pair of scissors, and used a pair of tweezers to pull out the retina. However, in spite of this laborious undertaking, he was not able to demonstrate the red colour of the retina until more than half a dozen animals had been killed. This unexpected result must have been of great concern.

Yet, five months later, in November 1876, the reason for the failure became apparent. He had discovered that the red colour of the retina in living animals was bleached in daylight and reappeared in darkness – before his demonstration in June 1876, the frogs had been kept in medium daylight (see Boll, 1877).

Furthermore, he discovered that the bleaching and regeneration of the red photopigment occurred in all animals with a retina containing rods; in cold-blooded and warm-blooded, vertebrates and invertebrates. Moreover, by using microscopy he found that the red colour was situated in the outer segment of the rods.

After these epoch-making discoveries, he could conclude that the red photopigment of the retina (later termed *visual purple* or *rhodopsin*) had to play an important role in visual processing. In his own words,

Diffuses Tageslicht macht die Purpurfarbe der Netzhaut erblassen. Längere Einwirkung directen Sonnenlichtes (Blendung) entfärbt die Retina vollständig. In der Dunkelheit stellt sich die intensive Purpurfarbe alsbald wieder her. Diese objective Veränderung der Aussenglieder durch die Lichtstrahlen bildet unstreitig einen Theil des Sehactes (Boll, 1877, p. 787).

(Diffuse daylight bleaches the red colour of the retina. When dazzling sunlight strikes the retina directly for long periods it becomes completely bleached. In the dark, the intense red colour quickly returns. These objective changes of the outer segments by light undoubtedly constitute a part of the visual process.)

In his paper, Boll (1878) demonstrated that different wavelengths differed in their ability to bleach the photopigment: red light had little or no effect, green-yellow light had a medium effect, while blue and violet lights had the strongest bleaching effect. This finding led him to speculate that the photochemical reactions of rhodopsin might furnish a basis for colour vision: wavelengths with the strongest bleaching effect might generate violet, wavelengths with medium bleaching effect green, while wavelengths with the smallest bleaching effect might generate a red sensation – all in harmony with the Young-Helmholtz colour theory.

Boll (1878) also found that frog retina contained yet another photopigment located in the outer segment of about 10% of the rod receptors. This pigment appeared green-blue and was also bleached in light and regenerated in the dark. He could not decide, however, whether this photopigment was a photoproduct of rhodopsin, or whether there were two different kinds of photopigment in the frog retina.

3.6 KÜHNE: SEVERAL PHOTOCHEMICAL SUBSTANCES IN THE RETINA

Immediately following Boll's discovery of the photochemical reaction of rhodopsin, Kühne (1877a, b, 1877–1878, 1879) made a very extensive investigation of this pigment. He accepted Boll's general view that visual sensations depended on photochemical processes, i.e. the initial reaction in the retina is the absorption of light by a photochemical see-substance. However, the speculation of Boll (1878) that the photochemical reaction of rhodopsin might constitute the basis for colour vision was rejected, since he found no rhodopsin in the human central fovea, where colour vision is best developed (Kühne, 1877a, p. 32, 1877b, p.107). In fact, he found no rhodopsin in cones, despite extensive investigations in different species including snakes, in which the retina contained only the cone receptor type (Kühne, 1877b, 1879).

Consequently, Kühne drew the conclusion that there had to be several photochemical substances in the retina, not just rhodopsin. Indeed, he suggested that the rod receptors, like the cones, contained colourless photochemical substances that could promote vision under conditions where the rhodopsin had been completely decomposed (Kühne, 1879, pp. 329–332). He found supporting evidence in that animals (rabbits) apparently with a pure rod retina could see even when rhodopsin had been bleached away.

Yet, in harmony with Schultze's duplicity theory, Kühne suggested that rhodopsin in rods represented the photopigment of twilight vision, only giving rise to achromatic sensations. Thus, he stated 'dass wir mittelst des Purpurs und der Stäbchen (ohne die Zapfen) das Spectrum nicht nur wahrnehmen, sondern auch in Grau schattirt, ähnlich wie der Farbenblinde, auffassen würden' ('that not only would we see the spectrum by means of the rhodopsin and the rods (without the cones) but also see it in shades of grey like the colour-blind'), and further,

Unsere Erfahrungen über das Vorkommen und Verhalten des Sehpurpurs sind so sehr in Uebereinstimmung mit M. Schultze's Hypothese von der physiologisch-chromatischen Bedeutung der Zapfen und Stäbchen, dass es nur des Hinweises darauf bedarf um alle Hoffnungen herabzustimmen, die man etwa auf die Optographie im Sinne specifischer Farbenwahrnehmung setzen mochte (Kühne, 1877a, p. 93).

(Our experiences of the occurrence and behaviour of rhodopsin are so highly consistent with M. Schultze's hypothesis about the physiological-chromatic impact of the cones and rods that one just needs to point to this experience in order to reject the hope that optography might have something to say about specific colour appeance.)

3.7 PHOTOTRANSDUCTION OF RHODOPSIN

Kühne also made an important contribution to our understanding of the transformation process of rhodopsin when activated by light. Thus, like Boll (1877), he found that rhodopsin first decomposed to a photoproduct that he called visual yellow (Sehgelb), and that this photoproduct further decomposed to yet another photoproduct, visual white (Sehweiss). Based on this finding, he made the important distinction between the photopigment (Sehstoff) and the photoproducts of the pigment (Sehreger) and suggested that it was the photoproducts that generated the neural activity in the retina (Kühne, 1879, p. 327).

Moreover, he discovered that rhodopsin may regenerate in two quite different ways: by a process which he named 'Anagenese' where the photoproducts visual white and visual yellow in the outer segment of the rods returned to rhodopsin and by another process which he called 'Neogenese' where rhodopsin, after having been completely bleached, was rebuilt by new substances (Kühne, 1879, pp. 317–323). The 'Anagenese' was assumed to proceed much more quickly than the 'Neogenese'. Hence, the speed of the dark adaptation process would be determined by the relative contribution of these two processes – complete bleaching would give the slowest recovery.

3.8 PARINAUD AND KÖNIG: EARLY
REFORMULATIONS OF THE DUPLICITY THEORY

Soon after the discoveries of Boll and Kühne, compelling new evidence in support of rhodopsin as the photochemical substance responsible for night vision was provided by Parinaud (1881, 1884b, 1885) and König (1894). On the basis of their discoveries they both presented their own version of the duplicity theory and have later been reckoned among its founders. We will, therefore, give an account of their contributions.

3.9 THE DUPLICITY THEORY OF PARINAUD

In harmony with Schultze's duplicity theory (1866), Parinaud assumed that the human retina contained two different types of photoreceptor, rods and cones, and that the cones gave rise to brightness, form and colour sensations, while the rods, being solely responsible for night vision, gave rise to achromatic sensation only. Also, under mesopic conditions, where rods and cones are activated simultaneously, the rod activity was assumed to influence both colour and form sensations by desaturating cone-mediated colours and increasing their brightness (like adding white light to a colour) and reducing acuity performance (Parinaud, 1885, p. 822).

In contrast to Schultze (1866), however, but in agreement with Newton (1675, 1730), Parinaud held that the essential cause of the different colour qualities had to be found in the brain and not in the optic nerve (Parinaud, 1884a, p. 242). Furthermore, he held that the rods were mediators of diffuse brightness sensation only.

Yet, his most important theoretical contribution, no doubt influenced by the remarkable discoveries of Boll and Kühne, was his far-reaching photochemical presumptions:

1. The initial light reaction of the rods is photochemical in nature, i.e. the nerve impulses are triggered by light acting on the photopigment rhodopsin. The initial light reaction of the cones, on the other hand, is of a physical nature (Parinaud, 1884b, 1885, p. 822).
2. Rhodopsin is broken down by light and regenerates in the dark. The amount of decomposition increases when the wavelength of the light stimulus decreases from red to blue, but then remains approximately constant in the violet part of the spectrum (Parinaud, 1884b).
3. The sensitivity of the eye increases with the amount of rhodopsin (Parinaud, 1885, p. 823).

With this last assumption, he explained both the sensitivity increase of the eye with dark adaptation and the sensitivity decrease with light adaptation, suggesting that only the rods, not the cones, adapted to changes in light levels (Parinaud, 1885, p. 823).

It appears that Parinaud arrived at his theory of rod and cone functions by his study of 'héméralopie' (note that in French 'héméralopie' means night blindness, while in English 'hemeralopia' means day blindness). By this term, he meant night blindness (in English 'nyctalopia') – a defect that reduces the sensitivity of the eye markedly. He explained this defect with the assumption that rhodopsin in the rods of the night blind was non-functioning (Parinaud, 1881). Thereby, the normal form and colour vision, and the lack of sensitivity increase during dark adaptation of the night blind could be accounted for. Moreover, he could explain the excellent acuity and colour discrimination within the rod-free fovea of humans and also the excellent acuity performance of pigeons and hens that lacked rhodopsin.

Furthermore, his photochemical presumptions could easily explain the change in size of the so-called photochromatic interval (the intensity interval between light and colour thresholds) obtained psychophysically in the extrafoveal retina in a dark-adapted state. Thus, in accordance with his predictions, the photochromatic interval was found to increase from the deep red to the blue part of the spectrum (bleaching effect increased) and to be absent when the measurements were made within the rod-free fovea.

Moreover, the deterioration of acuity performance observed when a test field is moved away from the central fovea (a major problem for Schultze) was accounted for by Parinaud with his assumptions that cones were the receptors responsible for form discrimination and that their number decreased with eccentricity (Parinaud, 1884a, p. 242, 1885, p. 822).

Finally, Parinaud (1884b) pointed out that his model also provided explanations for several other important psychophysical observations not adequately accounted for previously, e.g. the Purkinje phenomenon (see Purkinje, 1825) as well as difficulties encountered by photometric measurements. He did not formulate his arguments in any detail, however, probably because he found the explanations based on his model to be straightforward.

3.10 KÖNIG: RHODOPSIN IS THE MEDIATOR OF NIGHT VISION – A CONCLUSIVE PROOF

Parinaud's investigation of nyctalopia strongly indicated that rhodopsin was the photopigment responsible for night vision in humans. Even more compelling evidence in support of this suggestion was provided by König (1894). Using a spectrophotometer, he measured the absorption coefficient of the rhodopsin of the human eye over the spectrum from 640 nm to 420 nm and then compared the spectral absorption obtained with the spectral sensitivity measured psychophysically under scotopic conditions, in trichromats, dichromats and rod monochromats. The values of the two measurements corresponded excellently between 640 nm and 500 nm. Between 500 nm and 420 nm the spectral sensitivity was somewhat less than that calculated from the spectral absorption curve. This discrepancy could, however, be reasonably accounted for by the absorption of the macular and the lens pigments of the eye.

3.11 THE DUPLICITY THEORY OF KÖNIG

Having provided conclusive evidence that rhodopsin mediated night vision, König (1894) proceeded to formulate his special version of the duplicity theory by seven simple theses as stated below:

1. There is no visual purple in the central fovea or in any cone receptor. (The same conclusion had previously been reached by Kühne, 1877b, 1879.)
2. The colourless sensation obtained extrafoveally at the absolute threshold for all wavelengths (except for red-related wavelengths) is due to the decomposition of a small amount of rhodopsin.
3. Stronger decomposition of rhodopsin produces visual yellow, which is responsible for the primary blue colour sensation.
4. The unknown visual substances responsible for the 'red' and 'green' primaries are (like visual yellow) less sensitive to light than rhodopsin.

5. In total colour-blindness (i.e. rod monochromacy) there is no photopigment other than rhodopsin, and the visual yellow cannot be sufficiently decomposed by light to activate the primary blue sensation.
6. The Purkinje phenomenon and the breakdown of Newton's colour-mixture laws, found when the test intensity is increased, may be explained by the relative sensitivity change between rhodopsin and visual yellow. (In scotopic vision only rhodopsin may be activated by light and hence only achromatic sensations are obtained.)
7. The physiological process underlying 'white' sensation is not an increase of the process underlying the sensation of grey (die Grauempfindung).

The last thesis appears somewhat cryptic, but is probably intended to mean that two different processes underlie achromatic sensation: one generated by cones and the other by rods.

Theoretically, thesis 6 was most important, since it highlighted the limitation of the colour-mixture laws proposed by Newton (1730). From Newton's laws one would expect that when two lights match, with respect to hue, saturation and brightness, they would continue to match when the light level is proportionally reduced or increased, since the number of rays of each colour would change in the same proportion (see Grassmann, 1853; Helmholtz, 1855, p. 24).

The prediction that the match would hold when light intensity is changed also followed from the colour theory of Young-Helmholtz (Helmholtz, 1896). Clearly, quantum absorption of the three photopigments would be expected to remain equated when the intensity of two matched colour fields is reduced or increased in the same proportion.

Yet, late in the nineteenth century, the colour-mixture laws of Newton were found to break down under extrafoveal conditions (see von Kries, 1929). The additivity failure obtained could, however, be easily explained by the finding that the extrafoveal retina has four, instead of three, elementary receptor functions, and that only rhodopsin in rods may be activated in night vision. Thus, a colour match between a test and comparison field obtained in the extrafovea in a light-adapted state (i.e. under photopic conditions) would break down under mesopic and scotopic conditions if, under these conditions, the rod receptor system was not equally activated in the test and comparison fields.

König's third thesis is the most original one. It suggests, in opposition to both Schultze (1866) and Parinaud (1881, 1885), that rods may play an important role in colour vision. Previously, Ebbinghaus (1893) had speculated that the photopigments of rods could be identified as the yellow-blue substrate postulated by Hering (1878). Thus, the action of light on rhodopsin and visual yellow (a photoproduct of rhodopsin) was supposed to give rise to the sensation of yellow and blue, respectively. In agreement with Ebbinghaus, König (1894) assumed that the formation of visual yellow was necessary in order to obtain the primary blue sensation. Consequently, he held that the rod-free fovea was blue-blind. In opposition to Ebbinghaus, however, he suggested that activation of rhodopsin generated achromatic instead of yellow sensations – a suggestion based on his finding that light appeared achromatic, not yellow, under scotopic conditions where rhodopsin was responsible for vision.

In order to reconcile his assumption that visual yellow and rhodopsin situated in the same receptor generated two qualitatively different sensations with the specific fibre-energy doctrine, König (1894, p. 591) referred to complex processes originating in the sensorium. Other ways to explain this would have been to accept the ad hoc assumption of Helmholtz (1867) that different qualities may be transmitted through the same fibre or, alternatively, to presume that two different fibres, one subserving achromatic sensation, the other blue, were connected to each rod.

3.12 THE DUPLICITY THEORY OF VON KRIES

In contrast to Schultze, Boll, Kühne, Parinaud and König, von Kries (1894, 1896, 1911, 1929) did not provide compelling *new* evidence in support of the duplicity theory. Instead, he fulfilled the important role of promoting its general acceptance by presenting a comprehensive discussion of all available evidence in favour of the theory, including his own accurate experimental results (see von Kries, 1929).

Since von Kries was recognized as the leading authority on the duplicity theory, and the 1929 paper gives his final and most thorough defence of the theory, we will present this defence in some detail. The main evidence supporting the duplicity theory was discussed under three major headings:

1. *Lights that match in day vision may differ in twilight vision: the Purkinje phenomenon.*

Here, he presented experimental results which showed that a colour match between two light patches, obtained extrafoveally in a light-adapted state, may break down when the intensity of the two fields is lowered equally and the eye becomes dark adapted. Indeed, he showed that a colour match obtained in a light-adapted state at mesopic luminance levels may break down by dark adaptation without any change in light intensity.

As noted above, both of these observations were opposed to Newton's additivity law of colour mixture. With a suggestion similar to that of König (1894), von Kries explained the apparent additivity failure by the assumption that there were two different modes of vision, a chromatic day vision and an achromatic twilight vision, and that, as the mode of vision gradually changed from day vision to twilight vision, the colour field with the strongest twilight activation would gradually become relatively more desaturated and bright.

Obviously, this explanation implies that the two modes of vision may function simultaneously in an overlapping intensity range (the so-called mesopic intensity range), and that an increase of rod activity in a test field may reduce the saturation and increase the brightness of the test colour – all in agreement with Schultze (1866), Parinaud (1884b, 1885) and König (1894).

Strong support of the duplicity theory was also found in the observation that the breakdown of colour matches could be obtained in all parts of the extrafoveal retina, from the parafovea to the extreme periphery, but not in the central fovea where only cones were operating, and that only achromatic colours could be seen in twilight vision.

2. *Anatomical interpretation of the theory. Cones and Rods. Uniqueness of the fovea. Rhodopsin.*

Under this second heading, von Kries referred to a number of experiments which demonstrated the complete absence of the Purkinje shift in the rod-free foveal region. The evidence he found supported the suggestion that the cone receptors were the anatomical substrate of day vision, while the rods were the anatomical substrate of twilight vision. An even stronger argument in favour of this suggestion was the close relationship found between the spectral sensitivity of twilight vision and the degree of decomposition of rhodopsin with wavelength. Surprisingly, von Kries did not refer to König (1894), but to Trendelenburg, who much later obtained results similar to those of König (see von Kries, 1929, p. 691).

Lastly, the corresponding time between regeneration of rhodopsin and the sensitivity increase during dark adaptation measured extrafoveally (both processes take about 30 min to approach the final level) were mentioned as important evidence supporting the duplicity theory.

3. *Isolation of twilight vision. Congenital, total colour-blindness. Nyctalopia. On comparative anatomy.*

Here, under this third heading, von Kries presented experiments which showed that the spectral luminosity function in twilight vision was approximately the same and remained essentially invariant within the scotopic intensity range when measured in trichromats, dichromats and rod monochromats. In Fig. 3.1 the spectral sensitivity of rods and cones obtained at 30° extrafoveally are shown. As can be seen, the sensitivity difference between rods and cones is large in the short-wave and small in the long-wave region.

Finally, Schultze's observation that the relative number of rods to cones differed in the retina of diurnal and nocturnal animals, and the investigation of 'l'héméralopie' by Parinaud (1881), were found to support the duplicity theory.

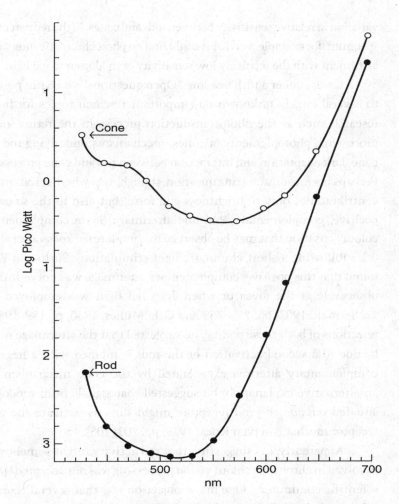

Fig. 3.1 Absolute spectral threshold curves obtained during the cone-plateau period (○) and in a completely dark-adapted eye (●) at 30° extrafoveally using a 1 × 2° test field exposed for 0.5 s.

The defence of the duplicity theory presented under these three headings represented von Kries's major arguments in favour of the duplicity theory, but under a fourth heading, 'Special items', he also pointed to several minor arguments. For instance, in accord with Parinaud (1884b), he emphasized that the variation of the size of the photochromatic interval with wavelength and with dark adaptation could easily be explained by variation in relative sensitivity between rods and cones. In the red part of the spectrum, for example, von Kries could find no photochromatic interval, in agreement with the relatively low sensitivity of rhodopsin to red light.

Lastly, under a fifth heading, 'Open questions', von Kries pointed to several largely unknown but important research topics for future research such as the phototransduction process in the retina, nerve processing, photopigments of cones, mechanisms underlying rod and cone dark adaptation and interaction between rod and cone processing. Perhaps his most interesting question, though, was whether rods might contribute not only to brightness and form, but also to the so-called positive, complementary Purkinje afterimage (i.e. a complementary colour sensation that may be observed in complete darkness after about 0.2 s following a short chromatic light stimulation). Since von Kries found that this positive, complementary afterimage was not ordinarily observable at the fovea or when deep red light was employed (see Tschermak, 1902, pp. 759–768 and G.E. Müller, 1930, pp.189–198 for rejections of both these points), he suggested that the afterimage might be due to a second activation of the rods combined with a negative complementary afterimage generated by the cone mechanism. As an alternative explanation, he suggested that signals from rhodopsin situated *outside* the rod receptors might directly activate the cone receptor mechanism (von Kries, 1929, pp. 702, 705).

Apparently, his suggestion that rod activity might somehow be involved in chromatic colour vision processing was not accepted by the scientific community. One major objection was that several research workers were able to obtain the Purkinje afterimage at the central fovea. (For alternative interpretations of the Purkinje afterimage, see Helmholtz (1911), p. 260; Tschermak (1902), pp. 759–768; and G.E. Müller (1930), pp. 189–198.)

3.13 AN ATTEMPT TO UNIFY THE THEORIES OF SCHULTZE AND YOUNG-HELMHOLTZ

In his 1929 paper von Kries mainly discussed the evidence already available in favour of the duplicity theory. In a previous paper he had made another important contribution by attempting to integrate evidence accumulated within the Newton and Schultze traditions into a unified theory (von Kries, 1911). In this endeavour he encountered a serious problem: no existing theory could adequately account for achromatic colour sensation. The explanation provided by the Young-Helmholtz colour theory had long been outdated. Clearly, the presumption that white sensation was generated by the three primary cone receptor types activated to about the same degree was challenged by the fact that the rod receptors also mediated achromatic sensation. Furthermore, it had been found that *monochromatic* spectral lights could give rise to colourless sensations under daylight conditions when the size of the test field was very small, and also when the test stimulus was exposed in the far peripheral retina (von Kries, 1911, pp. 430–432). Hence, a more comprehensive theory was called for.

In his attempt to provide a more adequate explanation of achromatic colour sensation, von Kries (1911) presumed that the white-related process could be provoked by two different *centrally* located mechanisms operating more or less independently of each other: the cone-related mechanism, with a tripartite structure, generating both chromatic and achromatic sensations; and the rod-related mechanism, with a unitary structure, reacting to different wavelengths in a qualitatively homogeneous manner, giving rise to achromatic vision only. Thus, day and night vision were thought to be special modes of vision based on separate and distinct parts of the visual organ as a whole (see von Kries, 1911, p. 395).

As revealed by the following quotation, however, von Kries was keenly aware of the fact that important problems remained to be solved, particularly with regard to the complex cone mechanism:

> ... it may be considered as extremely probable that the organisation in three components assumed in the Helmholtz theory does not apply to the organ of vision as a whole, but only to those parts that are directly exposed to the action of light and a more or less extended series of parts connected with them; and that, on the other

hand, the final results, the immediate substrata of the sensations, are themselves of a different nature; and hence that somewhere along the route the three independent results of stimulus are transformed into processes of a different kind and composition. As to these processes, nothing can be said with certainty, in the writer's opinion, except that in them the colourless sensation has some outstanding physiological significance (von Kries, 1911, pp. 431–432).

It will be seen that the duplicity theory offered by von Kries, like the Young-Helmholtz colour theory, had little to say about the actual neurophysiological colour processing beyond the receptor level. This ignorance is perhaps best illustrated by Helmholtz's (1896) final version of the Young-Helmholtz colour theory where he simply suggested that the colour-related processes from each receptor were independently transmitted to the brain through isolated nerve fibres.

4 The Goethe tradition: the phenomenological approach

4.1 PHENOMENOLOGICAL ANALYSIS MAY REVEAL UNDERLYING MATERIAL PROCESSES

The almost complete lack of knowledge about colour processing in the visual pathway is quite understandable. How could it be possible to obtain such information without microelectrodes or other advanced instruments at hand to monitor the processing?

An ingenious way out of this apparently insurmountable difficulty was offered by Hering (1878). He held that there were actually *two* quite different routes to understanding the processes underlying colour vision: a direct physiological approach and an indirect psychological approach. The psychological approach was based on the presumption that information about material processes underlying colour vision may be obtained by analyzing the phenomenological characteristics of colour sensations. Actually, Hering accepted the psychophysical maxim of Mach (1865, p. 320) that made three basic assumptions:

1. Every mental process is unalterably correlated with an underlying material process.
2. Similar and different mental processes are, respectively, correlated with similar and different material processes.
3. Every detail in the mental process corresponds to a detail in the material process.

As may be seen, the maxim of Mach is a specification of Spinoza's principle of psychophysical parallelism. It may also be noted that the maxim is akin to Leibniz's presumption that there is a pre-established conformity between mind and body (e.g. Boring, 1957, pp. 165–168).

Presupposing Mach's maxim to be valid, it would be a straight-forward undertaking to obtain information about material processes underlying colour sensation, once an unbiased and comprehensive phenomenological analysis of colour vision was worked out. By following this lead, Hering (1878) obtained strong evidence of opponent interactions between colour-related material processes and thereby challenged the basic assumption of the Newton tradition that no interaction between colour processes occurs in the visual pathway.

4.2 THE COLOUR THEORY OF J. W. VON GOETHE

Goethe (1810) had made a strong case for the phenomenological approach prior to Hering. Indeed, he had stressed the importance of a phenomenological analysis in its own right.

Apparently strongly influenced by the three leading German philosophers in the post-Kantian period, J. G. Fichte, F. W. J. von Schelling and G. W. F. Hegel, Goethe presumed that colour was an elementary phenomenon of nature that should be viewed in relation to other analogous phenomena like magnetism and electricity with the ultimate aim of uncovering the general laws of nature. He insisted that colour sensations should not be reduced to physiological processes, nor should they be represented by elementary, independent, physical units as Newton had done, but be regarded as *phenomena* in dynamic interactions with each other.

In order to obtain an adequate understanding of the basic processes governing colour appearance, he suggested that the whole range of colour phenomena should be explored, not just the very limited range investigated by Newton. He obtained an overview of the great variety of colour phenomena by dividing them into three different domains: colour phenomena primarily conditioned by (1) the visual system (e.g. afterimages), (2) colourless media (e.g. colours conditioned by prisms or clouds), and (3) properties of coloured objects (e.g. colours of the human skin). By exploring colour phenomena in these three domains closely, it would be possible, he believed, to reveal their basic laws (Goethe, 1810, Didaktischer Teil, pp. 21–294).

At the most fundamental level, Goethe presumed that light and dark, or as he also expressed it, light and not light, were polar or opponent phenomena and the prerequisite for all colour sensations. The most primitive and least developed colours were thought to be white and black. They were opponent and generated by light and dark, respectively. At a more advanced stage of development, he assumed that yellow may emerge when light is changed as a result of an interaction with dark, while blue may arise when dark is changed by an interaction with light. This development may proceed to higher levels. Thus, the yellow and blue colours, which were also thought to be opponent phenomena, may interact to generate a green colour. In fact, when the polarity between the two is in equilibrium, only pure green is observed with no trace of the yellow and blue components. Moreover, by gradually darkening or condensing yellow or blue, each of them would change towards red to such a degree that red eventually would dominate the colour appearance. Finally, a mixture of red-yellow and red-blue in due proportions would create the most highly developed colour – a pure red, which

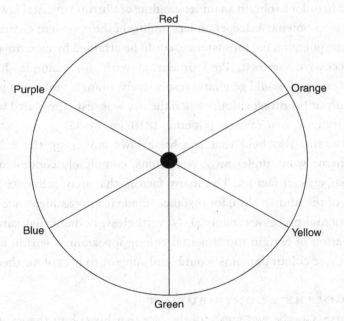

Fig. 4.1 Goethe's colour circle. The extremes of the diameter represent opponent colours. Note that the opponent colour of blue is orange and the opponent colour of yellow is purple.

Goethe termed 'Purpur' (Goethe, 1810, p. 228). Thus, in addition to the primitive white and black, Goethe acknowledged the development of six different basic colours and, of course, innumerable colours resulting from their combinations.

The colour theory of Goethe is best illustrated by his famous colour circle as shown in Fig. 4.1.

Thus, Goethe, like Newton, presented the different colour qualities on the circumference of a circle. The green colour was located between yellow and blue, violet between blue and red, and orange between red and yellow (Goethe, 1810, p. 287). Also, by a rotating diameter in the circle, he could determine all opponent colours by the two extremes of the diameter. Yet, in the final analysis, Goethe reduced all the opponent colours to three basic ones: yellow and red-blue; blue and red-yellow; pure red ('Purpur') and green (Goethe, 1810, p. 258).

Goethe stressed that one should perform the basic experiments oneself in order to obtain an understanding of the fundamental laws of colour phenomena. A deeper understanding of the opponent character of colour phenomena, for instance, could be attained by experiments on successive contrast. Pre-stimulation with, for example, blue, yellow or green would generate, respectively, orange, violet and pure red ('Purpur') contrast colours when the eye was test stimulated with an achromatic, neutral light (Goethe, 1810, pp. 44–45).

Goethe also held that the basic laws governing the colour phenomena were, under most conditions, completely concealed by more superficial factors. The many factors that may influence the colour of the human skin, for instance, made it impossible to see the fundamental processes involved. Nevertheless, he held that careful observation of certain fundamental colour appearances within each of the three colour domains would lend support to his colour theory.

4.3 GOETHE'S CONTRIBUTION

Of course, Goethe was aware of the fact that his colour theory was, to a great extent, a product of previous thinking. Thus, a concept of colour opponency had already, long ago been developed by Greek philosophers (e.g. Empedocles and Plato), and Aristotle had suggested that colour sensations could be generated by an interaction between white and black (Goethe, 1810, pp. 524–539). In fact, a colour theory similar to that of Goethe had previously been presented by Lazarus Nuguet (Goethe, 1810, pp. 748–756). Also, a serious limitation of his theory was the complete neglect of the physical and physiological basis of colour vision.

Yet, his historical review of colour theories (Goethe, 1810, Historischer Teil, pp. 513–986), his many experiments, his descriptions and analyses of a great variety of colour phenomena, his insistence on a phenomenological analysis of colour vision in its own right, even including the emotional characteristics of colours, and his concept of opponency, made a profound impact on later research within colour vision. The comprehensive work of Goethe made it quite clear that the observational basis of Newton had to be expanded in order to reach a more general understanding of the colour phenomena.

4.4 THE COLOUR THEORY OF EWALD HERING

Hering developed a new and ingenious colour theory by changing the basic presumptions of Goethe in two important ways (see Hering, 1878, 1964).

1. He proposed that the chromatic colours on the circumference of the colour circle should be ordered *quantitatively*. Thus, he presumed (a) that there are four primary hues, each of which reveals only one psychological quality: red, yellow, green or blue (this is in agreement with several other previous research workers, e.g. Aubert, 1865; Mach, 1865), and (b) that all the intermediate hues may be characterized by the relative distinctness of two of the primaries. Thus, all hues in the range between pure red and pure yellow, for example, may be characterized by the relative distinctness of red and yellow – the more similar the colour is to yellow, the less its similarity to red and vice versa. Accordingly, the colour series between pure red and pure yellow may be ordered quantitatively on the circumference of the circle by the ratio between the degree of similarity to red and

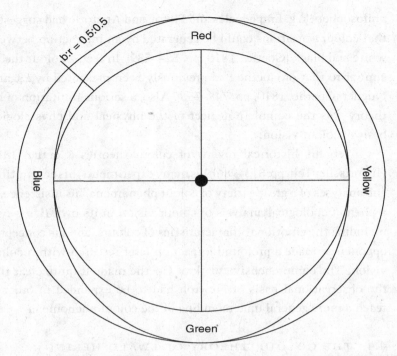

Fig. 4.2 Hering's colour circle. Note that, at variance with Goethe's colour circle, pure blue and pure yellow are opponent colours. The quantitative relationship between red and blue is illustrated for the case where $b/r = 0.5/0.5$. According to Hering's mathematical treatment it follows that $b = b/(r+b) = 0.5/1 = 0.5$ and $r = r/(r+b) = 0.5/1 = 0.5$.

the degree of similarity to yellow. Likewise, he assumed that the yellow-green, green-blue, blue-red and also the white-black series may be characterized, respectively, by the ratio between the degree of similarity to yellow and green, green and blue, blue and red, and white and black and, thereby, be treated in quantitative terms (see Fig. 4.2 for an illustration).

2. He accepted the psychophysical maxim of Mach (1865) and, hence, presumed that the analysis of the phenomenological character of colour sensations could give information with regard to the underlying material processes (Hering, 1878, pp. 70–77). The phenomenological analysis of the multiplicity of colour qualities had shown that they

could be expressed by six variables on whose relative proportion the different colour qualities would depend. From this finding and Mach's psychophysical maxim, Hering (1878) concluded that the correlated *material* processes could be expressed similarly, and that the quality of a colour directly correlated with the ratio of the magnitude of its underlying material process to the sum of all colour-related material processes operating simultaneously in the stimulated area. This sum, in turn, correlated with the impressiveness of the colour sensation. The green colour quality in a green-grey colour, for example, could be specified as $G/(G+W+B)$, that is, the magnitude of the material process underlying green relative to the sum of the material processes underlying green, white and black, while the impressiveness of the green-grey colour would correlate with the sum of the three different material processes $(G+W+B)$ (Hering, 1878, pp. 82–85). His quantitative analysis and mathematical treatment were rooted in what he termed 'das allgemeine psychophysische Grundgesetz' ('the common basic psychophysical doctrine'), particularly the maxim that the purity, plainness or clearness of a sensation depends on the ratio of the weight of the sensation to the sum of the weights of all simultaneously activated sensations (see Hering, 1878, p. 84).

The phenomenological analysis of the visible spectrum also revealed that there was no series of red-green or yellow-blue intermediate hues. That is, no hue in the spectrum appeared simultaneously red and green, or yellow and blue (Hering, 1964, p. 50). This mutually exclusive character of red and green, and of yellow and blue was also clearly displayed by binary colour mixtures where the two chromatic components either cancelled each other out completely or to the extent that only the dominant one was observed. Furthermore, the phenomenological analysis of the white-grey-black colour series revealed that white and black colour sensations were also opposed to each other. Thus, Hering could point to the fact that when white increased, black decreased and vice versa.

From these phenomenological analyses he concluded that the material processes underlying red, yellow and white were antagonistic to the material processes underlying, respectively, green, blue and black (Hering, 1878, pp. 70–126). Accordingly, he presumed that there were three pairs of opponent material processes: a 'red-green', a 'yellow-blue' and a 'white-black' pair, and that each pair had opposing metabolic dissimilation and assimilation processes in a 'see-substance' ('Sehsubstanz'). The red, yellow and white sensations were correlated with dissimilation processes that reduced the amount of the see-substance, while the green, blue and black sensations were correlated with assimilation processes that increased the amount of the see-substance. In the simplest version, the see-substance was assumed to consist of three different substances: a 'red-green', a 'yellow-blue' and a 'white-black' see-substance, where each could generate opposing dissimilation-assimilation processes independently of the activity of the other two. Hering did not locate these see-substances in the visual pathway. He simply suggested that waves of light in the ether generated chemical changes in the retina and that these changes triggered chemical processes in the optic nerve that eventually gave rise to chemical changes in the brain. Whether the see-substance was located only in the brain or also in the optic nerve and retina, he left undecided (Hering, 1878, pp. 70–75).

The 'red-green' see-substance could be activated by lights of all wavelengths, with the exception of pure yellow and pure blue, where the dissimilation and assimilation processes in the see-substance were assumed to be of equal magnitude, preventing any change in amount of substance. The same considerations also applied to the 'yellow-blue' see-substance, except that dissimilation and assimilation in this substance were assumed to be of equal magnitude for pure red and pure green light.

The 'white-black' see-substance, on the other hand, was assumed to differ from the two chromatic-related see-substances in two important respects: (1) the dissimilation and assimilation processes going on in this substance in darkness were assumed to be relatively large, and (2) light from the spectrum was assumed to only produce dissimilation in the stimulated area.

Interestingly, Hering speculated that if light could have activated the assimilation process in the 'white-black' see-substance, then the experience of black by such a light would have been much more intense than the most intense black we know of (Hering, 1878, pp. 88–89), and if a light stimulus could have produced equal dissimilation and assimilation in this substance alone, that light would have been invisible (Hering, 1878, p. 122).

A basic postulate in Hering's colour theory was his assumption that all six primary material processes were always in operation in all parts of the see-substance, despite the antagonistic actions of the dissimilation and assimilation processes (Hering, 1878, p. 85, pp. 118–120, and p. 126). The question then arises as to why red and green, and yellow and blue colours are mutually exclusive at the conscious level. Hering attempted to resolve this apparent paradox with his suggestion that dissimilation and assimilation in the 'red-green' and in the 'yellow-blue' see-substances had relatively low magnitudes and, hence, low impressiveness.

4.5 EXPERIMENTS IN SUPPORT OF HERING'S COLOUR THEORY

Besides the phenomenological analysis of the visual spectrum and the binary colour-mixture experiments, Hering found experiments on simultaneous and successive contrast, and simultaneous and successive induction, to be of particular importance in revealing information on the mechanisms of the underlying material processes (Hering,1878, pp. 95–103, 126–135). Thus, the experimental results he obtained could all easily be explained by the reasonable assumption that when one of the opponent processes was triggered by a light stimulus, the relative sensitivity of the antagonistic process increased with exposure time in the stimulated area and decreased in the neighbouring area.

As an illustration: when the eye, in a completely dark-adapted state, is pre-stimulated with a red light in a given retinal area (dissimilation increases) and, then, successively test-stimulated with an achromatic light in the same area, the achromatic light appears greenish. In this case, the green colour observed was explained by Hering in a straightforward manner by the assumption that the sensitivity of the 'red' dissimilation process compared to that of the 'green' assimilation process was reduced in the stimulated area during the pre-stimulation period.

4.6 CONTRIBUTIONS OF HERING

It can be seen that Hering agreed with Goethe that opponency is a fundamental characteristic of colour phenomena, but in addition he also postulated an opponency of underlying material events. This clearly opposes the suggestion of the Young-Helmholtz colour theory (1896) that the nervous pathways, from receptor to brain, are like isolated telegraph wires with no interaction between different neural processes.

With hindsight, we can see that Hering pointed in the right direction. Indeed, his ingenious ideas deserve to be ranked as *the fifth major paradigm shift in vision research*. Yet, his phenomenological approach has two serious weaknesses. Firstly, the phenomenological report gives conclusive information only on the *relative* values of the underlying material processes. In the case of the successive contrast experiment, for instance, where the red pre-stimulation produced a green after-effect upon test stimulation, Hering could reasonably presume that the sensitivity for dissimilation relative to that of assimilation was reduced in the red-green see-substance. But even if this presumption is accepted, he was not in a position to decide whether the sensitivity for assimilation in the test area increases or remains constant. The sensitivity might even decrease, although less so than for dissimilation (Hering, 1878, p. 86).

Secondly, presupposing that the psychophysical maxim of Mach (1865) is valid, one may draw legitimate conclusions about material processes directly underlying consciousness, but not about visual processes prior to the final material process. This limitation of the approach is clearly revealed when the conditions are arranged so that test stimulation of rods and cones initiates the same achromatic colour. Since the subject cannot discriminate between the achromatic colours obtained under photopic and scotopic conditions, it follows from the maxim of Mach that the underlying material events are the same. Hence, the researcher may be misled into neglecting the important retinal differences involved.

Of course, the finding that the rod and cone receptor systems may give rise to the same achromatic colour sensation was also a major challenge for the Young-Helmholtz trichromatic colour theory. Here, the white sensation was assumed to result from an equal stimulation of the three primary cone receptor systems, while the rod system did not have *any* significant role to play (see Helmholtz, 1867; von Kries, 1911).

These serious shortcomings of the Hering and Young-Helmholtz colour theories pointed to the need for a more comprehensive theory of colour vision where all the three major traditions were incorporated (i.e. the Newton, Schultze and Goethe traditions). This lead was followed by several research workers in the early 1900s. The most detailed and comprehensive theories were provided by Armin Tschermak (1902, 1929) and George Elias Müller (1896, 1897, 1923, 1930), both rooted in the Goethe tradition.

5   The colour theories of Armin Tschermak and George Elias Müller

5.1   THE COLOUR THEORY OF TSCHERMAK

In developing his own colour theory, Tschermak (1902, 1929) made a critical evaluation of the colour theories of Young-Helmholtz, Schultze and Hering. With regard to Young-Helmholtz's colour theory, he was severely critical. Thus, he asserted that the basic assumption of three independent, primary colour-related processes postulated by the trichromatic theory could not be reconciled with the phenomenological analysis of colour sensation that revealed *six* qualitatively different unitary sensations: red, yellow, green, blue, white and black. It would, for example, be impossible to give an adequate explanation of the uncompounded yellow-related material process by green- and red-related processes, or the uncompounded white-related process by red-, green- and violet-related processes. Also, in opposition to the trichromatic colour theory, experiments on colour mixture, colour induction and colour contrast clearly revealed opponent interaction processes going on in the visual system.

Finally, in accord with von Kries (1911), Tschermak (1902, 1929) pointed out that the basic assumption of the trichromatic colour theory, that white sensation was generated when the three different types of cone receptors were activated to about the same degree, was seriously challenged by the fact that colourless sensation could also be observed in scotopic vision where only rod receptors were known to function.

With regard to Schultze's duplicity theory, on the other hand, he found the evidence strongly in favour of its basic assumptions that cones functioned in day vision giving rise to both achromatic and chromatic sensations, and that rods functioned in night vision, giving rise to achromatic sensation only. He also accepted the basic assumption of Hering's opponent colour theory that colour vision rested upon independent, opponent 'red-green', 'yellow-blue' and 'white-black' material processes. On the basis of his evaluation, he came to the conclusion that there were five different kinds of cone receptor systems in the retina: an achromatic-, a red-, a yellow-, a green- and a blue-related system, in addition to the achromatic rod system.

Yet, his most original theoretical contribution was his suggestion that rhodopsin was situated not only in rods but also in small amounts in cones (Tschermak, 1929, p. 576). He found supporting evidence in the fact that several research workers had obtained the Purkinje phenomenon at the central fovea (Tschermak, 1902, p. 720). That some researchers (see e.g. von Kries, 1929) were unable to repeat this observation, he explained by the suggestion that the Purkinje phenomenon at the fovea was less pronounced than that obtained extrafoveally.

The suggestion of Tschermak that cones also contained rhodopsin raised the important question of how stimulation of rhodopsin might influence chromatic colour vision – a question discussed at length by G. E. Müller.

5.2 THE DUPLICITY THEORY OF G. E. MÜLLER

Along with von Kries, G. E. Müller was generally considered to be the leading authority in vision research in the 1920s. His colour theory was much more detailed and comprehensive than that of Tschermak (see G. E. Müller, 1896, 1897, 1923, 1930). It incorporated the basic knowledge of rod and cone functions accumulated up to 1930 and may be seen to represent the end of the first phase in the development of the duplicity theory, integrating evidence from the Newton, Schultze and Goethe traditions.

His theory, though, is highly speculative. Thus, in sharp contrast to the cautious theory construction of von Kries (1911), it gives detailed descriptions of colour processes in the visual pathway based on an almost complete lack of factual knowledge of the underlying neurophysiological processes. With hindsight, one may ask whether his far-reaching speculations have proved successful in promoting the development of the duplicity theory. Indeed, his theory may be seen as a test of the fruitfulness of providing comprehensive and speculative theories within vision research. In the following sections we present his theory in some detail.

5.2.1 G. E. Müller's speculation on the phototransduction in rods

In agreement with Kühne (1877a), Parinaud (1881, 1885), König (1894) and von Kries (1894, 1929), G. E. Müller held that rhodopsin was the photopigment of twilight vision and, consequently, that its spectral decomposition determined spectral sensitivity in a dark-adapted state at low test intensities (G. E. Müller, 1897, 1923). Also, he assumed that there was a continuous approach toward a state of equilibrium between decomposition and regeneration of the photopigment when it was acted upon by light.

At variance with Kühne, Parinaud, König and von Kries, however, he presumed that rhodopsin was but an optical sensitizer (optischen Sensibilisator). Its decomposition by light sensitized and, hence, increased the turnover of a base substance A ('Ausgangsmaterial') to a substance W ('W-material'). As the amount of this second substance increased, it was transformed into a third substance, substance V ('V-material'). The latter process, then (the change from the W to the V substance in the outer segment of the rods), was thought to be responsible for the 'white-' related neural activity ('W-Erregung') of the rods (G. E. Müller, 1923). An important and original consequence of this line of thinking was that rod sensitivity did not solely depend on the amount of rhodopsin, but also on the amount of the substance A available in the outer segment of the rod receptors.

5.2.2 Cones may inhibit regeneration of rhodopsin

In order to obtain a better understanding of how rod activity may change with light level, G. E. Müller (1923) made an extensive review of the available evidence concerning so-called rod monochromats.

He concluded that in a rod monochromat without functional cones, the rod receptors increased their activity as light level increased until at bright daylight the rod monochromat became dazzled and, hence, unable to discriminate any feature in the visual scene – seeing only a very bright, white light.

In the normal human retina, on the other hand, where both the rod and cone receptor systems are operative, the rod receptors were assumed to increase their output only up to a certain light level and, thereafter, to become increasingly inhibited by cone activity. The cone activity was assumed to inhibit the regeneration of rhodopsin and, thereby, reduce the rod output. Indeed, in bright daylight rhodopsin would not regenerate at all. Under this condition, there would eventually be no signals from rhodopsin to sensitize the 'A' substance and, as a consequence, this substance would regenerate to its dark-adapted value. Hence, the non-functioning of the rod system in bright daylight was assumed to be due solely to the lack of rhodopsin available in the rods.

Despite the inhibition from cones, however, rods were thought to operate at light levels several log units above the absolute dark-adapted cone threshold (e.g. in a room flooded with daylight) giving the possibility of simultaneous rod-cone activity over a long transitional intensity interval.

5.2.3 Rods subserving chromatic colour vision

G. E. Müller (1923) also made a thorough and noteworthy analysis of the available evidence of *chromatic* functioning of the rod system. The evidence procured was judged to indicate that decomposition of rhodopsin by light generated a weak green-blue colour sensation in addition to the prominent achromatic component. Yet, he could not decide, on the basis of the available evidence, whether the rhodopsin molecules responsible for the green-blue colour were situated in the outer segment of rods or cones. Evidence of a rod origin was found from colour sensations that were obtained by a rod-cone colour mixture under mesopic conditions and could be closely simulated by binocular colour mixture. G.E. Müller (1923) found this similarity consistent with a rod origin, since he assumed the rod and cone pathways were separated, perhaps to beyond the optic radiation, i.e. to the visual cortex.

The chromatic rod system would, of course, differ markedly from the chromatic cone system by operating at low light levels and subserving a green-blue colour invariant of wavelength. In order to explain the origin of such an odd chromatic rod system, G.E. Müller speculated that the rod system in a previous state of phylogenetic development, in fact, *could* discriminate between different coloured lights, but that the development of the photopigment rhodopsin, necessary for the increase of sensitivity during the second phase of long-term dark adaptation, was antagonistic to the formation of chromatic-related red-green and yellow-blue substances in the rods, so that only a primitive form of colour vision remained for the rod system.

5.2.4 Three types of cones and five pairs of opponent processes

The cone system, in contrast to the rod system, was assumed to have retained the ability to mediate the full range of colour sensations. In order to explain this marvellous ability, G.E. Müller made two basic assumptions: (1) the phototransduction in the retina, where light generates nervous activity, involved a triplex cone-receptor mechanism, and (2) colour processing was based on opponent activities. Accordingly, he considered both the Young-Helmholtz and the Hering colour theories to be over-simplifications (see foreword G.E. Müller, 1930).

A simplified diagram of his theory is shown in Fig. 5.1. For illustrative purposes, only activation of the rod and one of the three cone systems (P1) are shown. As can be seen, though, the difference between the rod and cone systems is marked. In fact, the rod system involves two white-black systems and possibly an undeveloped green-blue colour system, while the cone systems with photon-absorption processes P1 (sensitive from the extreme longwave end of the visual

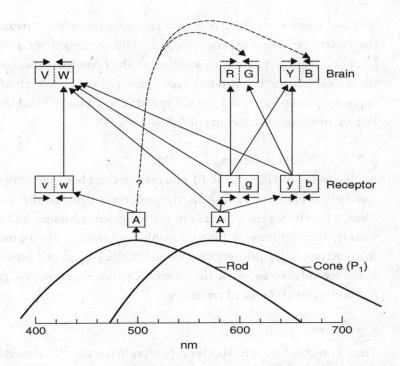

Fig. 5.1 A simplified illustration of G.E. Müller's duplicity theory representing only the rod and the P_1 cone systems. The P_1 cone absorbs light from the extreme long-wave end of the spectrum to about 475 nm, while the rod receptor contains rhodopsin and absorbs maximally at about 510 nm. 'A' represents the 'Ausgangsmaterial'. (v-w), (r-g) and (y-b) represent opponent processes in the outer segment of the receptors, while (V-W), (R-G) and (Y-B) represent opponent processes in the 'see-substance' (see text).

spectrum to about 475 nm), P2 (sensitive between 650 nm and 415 nm) and P3 (sensitive from about 540 nm to the extreme short-wave end of the visual spectrum) involve both a white-black and four pairs of chromatic opponent systems.

5.2.5   Activation of opponent processes by P1, P2 and P3

In harmony with Hering's colour theory, R-G, Y-B and W-V of Fig. 5.1 represent so-called 'see-substances' where red-green (R-G), yellow-blue

(Y-B) and white-black (W-S) opponent processes take place. To explain the variety of colour experiences, G. E. Müller needed yet another level of complexity. Thus, in addition to the opponent processes in the see-substances, he introduced red-green (r-g) and yellow-blue (y-b) opponent processes in a red-green (r-g) and yellow-blue (y-b) substance located in the outer segments of the cones.

5.2.6   The P1 system

As illustrated in Fig. 5.1, the P1 process activates both the red-green and yellow-blue substances in the outer segment of the cones. Thus, P1 activates the r-process in the red-green substance and also, weakly, the y-process in the yellow-blue substance. The r-process, then, activates red (R)-, yellow (Y)- and white (W)-related processes in the see-substances, while the y-process activates yellow (Y)-, green (G)- and white (W)-related processes.

5.2.7   The P2 system

The P2 process first activates the g-process in the red-green substance in the outer segment of the cones and the y-process in the yellow-blue substance. Then, the g-process activates the green (G)-, blue (B)- and black (S)-related processes in the see-substances, while the y-process activates the yellow (Y)-, green (G)- and white (W)-related processes like the y-process of P1.

5.2.8   The P3 system

Finally, the P3 process first activates the b-process in the yellow-blue substance in the outer segment of the cones and then the blue (B)-, red (R)- and black (S)-related processes in the see-substances. In addition to this complex processing, P1, P2 and P3 all directly activate the white (W)-related process.

Both the processes in the red-green and yellow-blue substances *in the outer segment* of the cone receptors and the processes in the see-substances were assumed to be of an antagonistic nature and to closely follow the same reaction pattern. They may, therefore, all be illustrated by G. E. Müller's model for the r-process in the red-green substance presented in the following simplified diagram:

Red light $\rightarrow$ photon-absorption process $P1 \rightarrow A \rightarrow r \rightarrow g$

As can be seen, red light activates P1 that increases the turnover of the base substance A to a substance r. As the amount of this second substance increases, it is transformed into a third substance g. The change from r to g generates the r-process, while the g-process is generated when the process goes in the opposite direction, from substance g to substance r. The r substance may then be transformed back to A.

This complex and highly speculative colour theory of the rod and cone systems may be seen as an attempt to cover all the major facts of colour vision available. The theory deviates markedly from both the Young-Helmholtz and the Hering colour theories. At variance with the Young-Helmholtz theory, it involves both opponent colour processing and rod activity, while in opposition to Hering's theory, it involves rod activity and operates with a triplex photochemical cone mechanism. Moreover, in contrast to Hering, who assumed the so-called 'Urfarben' (pure red, pure yellow, pure green and pure blue) to be correlated with homogenous, uncompounded material processes, G. E. Müller (1930) assumed that these colours were determined by complex processes in the outer segments of the cones. A *pure yellow colour* of the Hering type, for example, would be determined by both P1 and P2 and, hence, by r-, y- and g-processes in the outer segment of the cone receptors.

5.3 EVALUATION OF G. E. MÜLLER'S COLOUR THEORY

With hindsight, it seems clear that G. E. Müller's broad speculation on the actual colour-related processes in the visual pathways, based on insufficient evidence, did not entail a new, deeper understanding of rod and cone functions. Indeed, alternative theories that explained the same colour phenomena equally well were developed. An interesting example is the colour theory presented by Schjelderup

(1920). In addition to the processing put forward by G. E. Müller, Schjelderup postulated a stage of colour processing in the cortex where six independent physiological processes (red-, yellow-, green-, blue-, white- and black-related processes) operated. By further assuming that each of these independent chromatic processes of the cortex could be lacking or non-functioning, he held that he could explain the different types of colour-blindness better than G. E. Müller (see Schjelderup, 1920).

Even though the speculations of G. E. Müller did not provide important new information about colour processing, they revealed the lack of factual knowledge available and, thereby, stressed the need for the development of new instruments and techniques designed to map the anatomical details of neural elements, and to monitor *actual* biochemical and physiological processes. The next developmental period of the duplicity theory from 1930–1966 met this need.

Part II The development of the duplicity theory from 1930–1966

In this developmental period, profound new knowledge about the anatomical and neurophysiological properties of the retina emerged as a result of advances in sophisticated instrumentation and research techniques. This knowledge greatly influenced the development of the duplicity theory: it provided an insight into the rod and cone processes, and also created and paved the way for new ideas of rod and cone functioning. Outstanding contributions to the development were provided by Polyak, Hartline, Kuffler and Granit. Using the Golgi impregnation method, Polyak's investigation of the primate retina helped to elucidate the extremely complex structure of the many types of retinal cells and the character of their connections. Hartline, Kuffler and Granit, using microelectrodes for registration of the action potential from individual nerve fibres in response to illumination, increased our knowledge about the relationship between light stimuli and nerve impulses in the retina.

6   The duplicity theory of Polyak

After a comprehensive review of the anatomical and histological research on the organs of vision from the classical antiquity to his own time, Polyak (1941) concluded that this research had played a relatively insignificant role in forming hypotheses and theories of the *function* of the visual system. A major reason was that the retina of humans and other primates had never been examined in any detail by analytical histological methods such as those of Golgi and Ehrlich. These methods, although very time consuming, were preferable, since they permitted the staining of only a few nerve cells at a time from the bewildering mass of tissues. Indeed, in successfully treated preparations, the individual neurons could be stained completely, revealing the whole nerve cell with all its extensions and branches extending as far as the finest terminals. Furthermore, he held that a disclosure of the structural details of the retina of primates would make possible interpretations related to the many psychophysical functions already established in humans.

Polyak, therefore, completed a very impressive histological investigation on the retina of macaques and chimpanzees, using the Golgi method. He also occasionally used retinas from humans. His comprehensive and seminal research work (summarized in 1941; second impression, 1948) has long been recognized as a classic contribution to our knowledge of the retinal structure and function in primates.

His results confirmed two of the basic findings of Schultze (1866): (1) the retina of primates contained two morphologically clearly differentiated varieties of photoreceptors, the rods and cones, and (2) the structure of cones did not differ essentially within any of the retinal regions. They all appeared to belong to the same variety, possessing the same structure and synaptic relationships. Polyak, therefore, like Schultze, presumed that they were functionally equivalent.

Yet, Polyak found that the cone receptors in *different* regions of the primate retina had somewhat different structures and that they, therefore, probably also differed somewhat with regard to function. Thus, Polyak held that the cones in the foveal centre were farthest advanced in their structure and biochemical differentiation and capable of the most elaborate and diverse responses, and that the responses gradually became more crude and summary in character as the ora serrata was approached.

6.1 TRICHROMACY OF COLOUR VISION EXPLAINED BY THREE TYPES OF BIPOLAR CELL

Schultze had explained trichromacy, demonstrated by Maxwell (1860), by suggesting that different spectral lights affected different outgoing fibres connected to the inner segment of each cone in a qualitatively different manner. Polyak, however, did not agree with Schultze that the mechanism of trichromacy was located in each cone receptor. Using the Golgi technique, he could find no evidence of three distinct varieties of minute structures or organelles that could serve as chromatic analyzers in the cone receptors of primates. He therefore, at variance with Schultze, presumed that the cone response, over short time intervals, was rather uniform and homogeneous, spreading over the entire cone cell, including all its extensions. To explain the close connection between wavelength of light and hue sensation, he suggested that at different times the photosensitive cone substance would generate different kinds of dynamic changes subserving different kinds of colour sensations when activated by different wavelengths or different wavelength combinations.

But if each cone may mediate hundreds of different kinds of uniform colour-related reactions in response to different wavelengths, then how could the trichromacy of colour vision be explained? Obviously, the numerous colour-related cone excitations had to be reduced to three basic processes somewhere in the visual pathway.

Polyak pointed to the bipolar cells as promising candidates for performing this analyzing function. These neurons were positioned between the cones and the ganglion cells and therefore had to be regarded as the sole centripetal transmitter of the cone impulses. Also, Polyak had found the number of bipolar cell types in the primate retinas corresponded closely to the number of fibres postulated by the three-component theory of Young (1802). Polyak named four varieties: the mop, brush, flat and midget bipolar, but was uncertain whether the brush and flat bipolar cells actually represented different types.

To explain their analyzing functions, Polyak suggested, as the most probable hypothesis, that although each bipolar variety had preserved its original universal responsiveness to the visual spectrum, to some extent, each of them had become especially responsive to a particular part of the spectrum. Presuming that the cones had their maximum sensitivity in the long-wave region of the spectrum, Polyak suggested that the midget bipolar cells, being exclusively connected to cones, were chiefly responsive to cone impulses corresponding to this spectral region, while they were moderately responsive to the middle region, and least, if responsive at all to the short-wave region. The responsiveness of the mop bipolar cells, on the other hand, was assumed to be just the reverse, since he had discovered that this bipolar variety was chiefly connected to the rods that were known to be most sensitive to relatively short wavelengths. Finally, the brush and flat bipolar cells were assumed to be chiefly concerned with transmission of impulses corresponding to the middle part and less so to the two ends of the spectrum. As can be seen, Polyak made use of three types of bipolar cell, instead of three types of cone, to satisfy the requirement of the three-component theory.

The next problem confronting Polyak was to account for the apparent synthesis of the different colour-related processes. Obviously, since mixing the three primaries may produce colour sensations that are appreciated as a single quality, some merging and combination of the visual responses have to take place subsequent to the analyzing process.

6.2 MIDGET GANGLION CELLS AS SYNTHESIZERS

Polyak's histological investigation had revealed that the retina of primates had a very complex neural structure. This finding challenged the validity of the basic presumptions of Schultze's (1866) and Helmholtz's (1896) colour theories that the three different kinds of colour-related processes were transmitted independently from the photoreceptor to the brain, where eventually the integration processing took place. Indeed, Polyak's investigation of the structural details of the retina made evident that the ganglion cells were probably as essential for the transformation of the centripetal dynamic visual current as the bipolar cells. Thus, after passing through the bipolar cells, the impulses generated in the photoreceptors were found to be transmitted by *five* different varieties of ganglion cells before they were conveyed to the brain. Presuming that the bipolar cells were analyzers, Polyak came to the conclusion that the synthesis and compounding of the transmuted cone impulses, at least partially, were carried out by the ganglion cells of the retina. Furthermore, by an examination of the morphological features, especially the synaptic characteristics of the different types of ganglion cells, Polyak found reason to believe that only the midget ganglion cells could carry out the synthesis of the three primary colour-related excitations into compound processes. This was because of their relatively great number and small size, and because only the midget ganglion cells were related to all varieties of amacrine cells. He found additional evidence in support of his assumption in psychophysical studies which showed that in the centre of the field of vision, corresponding to the area of highest acuity, the smallest discernible object could be seen in variously coloured lights rapidly following one another, and also that it was impossible to observe two different colours simultaneously at the same location.

6.3 THE SPECIFIC FIBRE-ENERGY DOCTRINE QUESTIONED

Polyak concluded that each midget ganglion cell had the ability to transmit to the brain the entire range of spectral colour-related impulses received from the three or four different kinds of bipolar cells. This presumption, of course, clearly violated the specific fibre-energy doctrine of Helmholtz (1896) and also appeared to be in conflict with electrophysiological recordings from single nerve fibres where only one kind of electrical activity had been recorded (Graham & Hartline, 1935). In opposition to the doctrine of Helmholtz, however, Polyak stressed the possibility that the mode of reaction of a nerve fibre might be 'plastic'. Thus, he suggested that a great variety of bioelectrical and chemical processes of different kinds might take place in the neuro-plasma of a nerve fibre while eliciting substantially the same outward electrical manifestation registered by the microelectrode. Different qualities might also be coded by special groupings of the impulses in time, for example, by rhythmical groupings not yet known. Furthermore, in defence of his colour theory, Polyak pointed to the fact that the retina had a very complex structure and was made up of basically the same nerve cells as found in the brain, where evidently different qualities could emerge. He did admit, however, that little was yet known with regard to the ability of the same neuron or nerve fibre to generate and to conduct different modalities and qualities of dynamical changes.

6.4 APPLICATIONS OF POLYAK'S COLOUR THEORY

Polyak held that his colour theory, because of its general character, was applicable to a number of other colour theories in addition to Young's trichromatic colour theory. The basic requirements of Hering's opponent colour theory, for example, could be satisfied by the assumption that transmission of each dissimilation- assimilation process (the red-green, yellow-blue and white-black antagonistic processes) was carried out by one of the three bipolar varieties.

Furthermore, Polyak argued that his colour theory provided new insight into the material causes of various forms of colour-blindness: protanopia, deuteranopia, tritanopia, various forms of anomalous trichromatism, monochromatism, and also partial and complete blindness. Instead of failures of cones, one, two or all three types of bipolar cell might be absent or somehow impaired, or they might be incompletely differentiated into clear-cut types. Without bipolar cells the visual impulses from cones would be blocked and complete blindness would result.

6.5 COMMON PATHWAYS OF RODS AND CONES

Polyak's histological investigation of the primate retina also resulted in profound new insights into the function of the rod system. Schultze (1866) had presumed that the rod impulses were transmitted independently of the cone impulses to the brain. Strong supporting evidence had been provided by Ramon y Cajal (1937). Presuming, like Schultze, that there were two fundamentally different receptor types, rods and cones, that functioned under quite different conditions mediating qualitatively different colour sensations, Cajal predicted that there had to be two different types of bipolar cell in the retina: those connected solely to rods and those connected solely to cones. Indeed, he assumed that there had to be separate rod and cone pathways all the way from the photoreceptors to the brain (see Cajal, 1937, p. 384, Fig. 47 and pp. 393–395). In accord with his prediction, Cajal, in a series of histological studies on both fish and mammals, found that the rod and cone receptors were connected to different types of bipolar cell.

Polyak (1948), however, strongly rejected Cajal's idea that the rod and cone impulses travelled along separate routes to the brain. In fact, he found that all the bipolar and ganglion cell varieties, except the midget bipolar variety that was exclusively connected to the cones, were common to both the rod and cone systems. By examining Cajal's own histological results, he also pointed out that these results indicated common rod and cone pathways, since the rod bipolar cells shown could scarcely avoid contact with cone pedicles, at least in the central region of the retina. Indeed, Cajal, in an earlier paper, had suggested that the rod and cone pathways to the bipolar cells were not completely separated from each other, but that each pathway was dominated by either rod or cone impulses (see Cajal, 1894, p. 129).

Polyak's arguments prevailed, but his conclusion raised the important question of how rod impulses that mediated achromatic sensation, irrespective of wavelength, and cone impulses that mediated more than a hundred different hue sensations dependent on wavelength, could be transmitted through the same neural pathway. Polyak presented several solutions to this problem:

1. Since rods and cones may function under different conditions, the two receptor systems might use the common pathway at different times. Accordingly, Polyak suggested that, for example, the mop bipolar cells might mediate achromatic colour sensation in scotopic vision, while in photopic vision they might mediate bluish colours.
2. Rod impulses in photopic vision might be excluded from the common pathway by being inhibited either at the rod-bipolar synapse or in the bipolar cells themselves by the passage of the cone impulses.
3. Under conditions where the two receptor systems were activated simultaneously and both transmitted impulses to the brain, for example during the transition from photopic to scotopic vision or vice versa, there would be no serious problem as long as the impulses from the rods and cones both subserved achromatic colours and hence could be assumed to represent the same biophysical process. For conditions where the rod and cone impulses subserved different colour qualities, the rods achromatic, the cones chromatic sensation, Polyak offered several alternative solutions: (a) the different qualities might fuse into one entity, (b) the rod and cone impulses might alternate in time, (c) the cone impulses could be partly identical to the rod impulses and partly made up of other components different from and superimposed upon the rod activity, and (d) the mop bipolar cells alone might 'pick' the impulses common to both the rods and cones, whereas the other diffuse bipolar cells (brush and flat) and the midget bipolar cells might receive impulses predominantly or exclusively from the cones, each variety of bipolar cell 'picking' its own peculiar quality.

Polyak held that these and similar possibilities should be tested out by experiments before any firm and valid functional interpretation of the common pathways could be decided on.

6.6 EXPLANATIONS OF ACUITY AND SENSITIVITY DIFFERENCES BETWEEN RODS AND CONES

Schultze (1866) in his formulation of the duplicity theory could give no adequate explanation of the difference in acuity performance obtained psychophysically between the rod and cone receptor systems. Since the rod receptors were closely packed, more slender and also much more numerous than the cones, Schultze had expected, contrary to the facts, that rods would generally show better acuity performance than the cones.

A solution to this paradox was found when the Golgi method was introduced to reveal fine structural relationships in the retina. Thus, the histological investigations of both Cajal and Polyak revealed that the rod system was arranged in spatially larger functional units than the cone system. Polyak's investigation was the most important one, since he investigated retinas of primates and also discovered the so-called midget cone system, i.e. a monosynaptic relationship between cones and bipolar cells and between bipolar and ganglion cells, affording a 'private' conducting cone system in the central fovea of the primate. Polyak held that such a system would be best suited to serve as a mechanism for the most delicate space resolving and localizing functions. Its degree of refinement would depend on the cone gradient only and, hence, peak in the centre of the fovea.

A complication was introduced in that the midget system was strictly monosynaptic only in the central foveal region becoming gradually coarser out towards the orea serrata, since polysynaptic connections increased collecting impulses from several cones into the functional units. Hence, acuity would no longer depend on cone gradient alone, but also upon the synaptic relations of the midget system.

The reason for the relatively low acuity performance of the rod system was clearly revealed when Polyak showed that in the central part of the retina several rods were connected to a functional unit and that the rod system, even more than the midget cone system, displayed an increasing coarsening of the functional unit from the foveal region towards the orea serrata. Thus, he could provide explanation both for Schultze's paradox of the observed acuity difference between the rod and cone systems, and the decrease in acuity performance with eccentricity.

The structural arrangement and synaptic connections of the primate retina shown by Polyak by the Golgi method also provided new insight into the light *sensitivity* difference between the rod and cone systems. Since many more rods than cones were connected to a given functional unit, more rod impulses could be combined and, thereby, make the rod system the most sensitive. Hence, photochemical differences between the cone and rod receptor type could no longer be regarded as the sole explanatory factor of the greater rod sensitivity.

6.7 THE FUNCTIONAL POTENTIALS OF THE SYNAPTIC ARRANGEMENT

Even more important, the histological investigation of the retina with the Golgi method revealed that the retinal neural tissue was not composed of intimately related neurons in *continuous* nerve nets or nerve webs, but was made up of individual nerve cells only in contact with each other through synapses. This profound insight into the structure of the neural system had been revealed by Cajal in the late 1880s (see Cajal, 1937), but it was not until Polyak (1941) published his great work that the full functional potential of the primate retina became apparent. Thus, Polyak revealed that the neural structure of the primate retina was much more complicated than previously held. Both the bipolar and ganglion cells were composed of several varieties woven into an intricate synaptic pattern. Such a structure, of course, made possible much more varied reactions than a neuron network or neuron web composed of neurons of the same or similar kinds. In particular, Polyak pointed to the possibility that the location and number of synaptic contacts might affect both the kind and magnitude of an input received by a neuron, and that horizontal and amacrine cells might be involved in facilitation and inhibition of the centripetal impulses. Also, he stressed the interesting possibility that the output reactions of a given neuron, both with regard to quantity and quality, might depend not so much upon the input as upon its own innate disposition, as illustrated by the *bioelectrical* output of the photoreceptors elicited by the *light* energy input.

Polyak's theory of rod and cone functions, although highly speculative, was based on far more accurate histological data than the theory of Schultze. His results strongly indicated that some of the basic assumptions of Schultze had to be reformulated. Thus, he could find no evidence of three distinct varieties of minute structures that could serve as chromatic analyzers in the cone receptors and also showed that several of the bipolar and ganglion cell varieties were connected to both the rod and cone systems. Indeed, Polyak's own functional interpretation of the histological structure of the retina of the primate made it seem possible that colour vision, sensitivity regulation and acuity performances to a large extent were controlled by bipolar, horizontal, amacrine and ganglion cells and their synaptic relations.

Milestones in the further development of our understanding of the function of rods and cones are represented by the works of H. K. Hartline, S. W. Kuffler and R. Granit.

7 Investigations of H. K. Hartline and S. W. Kuffler

Newton (1675) had rightly presumed that light signals were transformed in the retina, and that the information about the visual world was conveyed to the brain by the optic nerve. His suggestion that visual information was transmitted by a vibration code, however, proved to be wrong. Thus, early in the twentieth century it had become generally accepted that the optic nerve fibres reacted to light by discharging a series of brief electrical action potentials. With increasing light intensity, the fibres tended to increase their firing rate, but the size of the discharge remained constant. (For a review of how our knowledge about the electrical nature of nerve impulses emerged, see Boring, 1957, pp. 30, 39–43 and Granit, 1947.)

7.1 THE ELECTRICAL RESPONSES TO LIGHT STIMULI IN SINGLE OPTIC NERVE FIBRES

H. K. Hartline was the first to make a thorough investigation of the electrical responses to light stimuli in single optic nerve fibres. A small bundle of fibres dissected from the optic nerve was split successively until only a single fibre remained. Thereafter, the electrical activity of the fibre, generated by a light stimulus, was recorded by means of an oscillograph capable of registering small, rapid voltage fluctuations. The recordings were made under conditions where the eye was illuminated by light of various intensities, durations and wavelengths (see Hartline, 1940, for a review).

7.2 THE ELECTRICAL RESPONSES IN SINGLE OPTIC NERVE FIBRES OF *Limulus*

In the retina of *Limulus* (horseshoe crab), where each photoreceptor is directly linked with a separate nerve fibre, Hartline found that a brief flash of light after an appreciable latency period caused a discharge of impulses in the fibre which lasted for several seconds. The total number of impulses elicited and the discharge frequency were found to increase with the intensity of the flash. These findings were in accord with what might be expected. Surprisingly, however, Hartline found that the magnitude of each impulse discharge was the same when intensity or duration of the light stimulus was varied. Also, he found that different test wavelengths could be made to evoke the same frequency of impulses from a given receptor cell by adjusting the incident light energy (Graham & Hartline, 1935). On this evidence the authors concluded that single receptors were unable to discriminate between wavelength and intensity, a characteristic of receptors later termed 'the Principle of Univariance'. This principle implies that at least two different types of photoreceptor must be present in the retina in order to distinguish between different colour qualities of different wavelengths.

With exposure of short duration, Hartline found, in accord with the reciprocity law of photochemistry (the Bunsen-Roscoe law), that the response pattern of the nerve fibre did not vary as long as the total amount of light energy (light intensity multiplied with duration) remained constant, strongly suggesting that the phototransduction process was photochemical in nature. Based on this suggestion he could determine the absorption spectrum of the photosensitive substance of single receptors in *Limulus* (responsible for excitation of a single optic nerve fibre) simply by measuring the reciprocal of the relative light energy of different wavelengths needed to produce a specific burst of impulses (Graham & Hartline, 1935).

The impulse pattern obtained from single optic nerve fibres of *Limulus* was also found to be affected by light and dark adaptation. Thus, during light adaptation the frequency of the discharge of impulses from single nerve fibres of a light stimulus declined to a steady level, while it showed a progressive recovery during dark adaptation.

Hartline (1940) ascribed the decline and recovery of the frequency of impulses to depletion and regeneration of the photosensitive substance of the receptors. Furthermore, he explained the steady discharge of impulses recorded after light adaptation had stabilized on the assumption that the rate of decomposition and regeneration of the photosensitive substance had reached a state of equilibrium.

7.3 THE ELECTRICAL RESPONSES IN SINGLE OPTIC NERVE FIBRES OF THE FROG

Hartline also made use of cold-blooded vertebrate frog retina in his investigation. In accord with his results on *Limulus*, the frequency of discharge in different fibres was found to be greater the higher the intensity of the retinal illumination, and it could be reduced and increased by light and dark adaptation. However, while the response pattern in nerve fibres of *Limulus* was found to be essentially similar in character, Hartline found three quite different response patterns in the frog retina:

1. In some fibres (so-called 'on' fibres) the discharge was similar to that of *Limulus*; the impulses were discharged regularly as long as the light was on.
2. Other fibres ('on-off' fibres) discharged impulses briefly when the light was turned on and again when it was turned off with no activity in between.
3. A third category of fibres ('off' fibres) discharged impulses only when the light was turned off.

This diversity of response was ascribed to the complex nervous structure interposed between the receptor elements and the ganglion cells of the frog retina.

An interesting feature of the impulses in the 'off' fibres was their strong suppression by re-illumination. This phenomenon was interpreted to mean that excitation of nerve cells may inhibit nerve activity. Hartline also found the 'on-off' fibres of the frog retina to be extremely sensitive to movements of retinal images: the more rapid and more extensive the movement, the greater the number of impulses at 'on' and 'off'.

Moreover, exploring the retina of the frog using a small spot of light, Hartline found that the receptive field of a ganglion cell (defined as the area of the retina which when illuminated may cause a discharge in the particular ganglion cell, i.e. the retinal region occupied by photoreceptors whose connections converge upon the ganglion cell) was maximally sensitive in the centre of the field, and that the sensitivity gradually fell off with increasing distance from this centre. Also, when the area of the receptive field illuminated was increased, the response of the ganglion cell increased, demonstrating spatial summation in the retina of the frog. Clearly, several retinal pathways had to converge upon the ganglion cell producing a combined effect.

7.4 RECEPTIVE FIELD ORGANIZATION OF RODS AND CONES: KUFFLER'S INVESTIGATION

The investigation of Hartline was followed up by Kuffler (1953). He made an extensive study of the configuration and functional organization of receptive fields in the retina of cats. Discharge patterns of single ganglion cells of the cat retina were recorded with a microelectrode while light stimuli were applied to different areas of its receptive field. Two small independently controlled light beams and also a background light field that determined the adaptation level of the retina were employed.

With this technique, Kuffler (1953) obtained several very interesting results. He showed that the retina contained receptive fields with central and peripheral areas that had opposite discharge patterns. Fields with 'on'-centre regions had 'off' surrounds and vice versa. In intermediary regions between the central and peripheral areas 'on-off' response patterns could be recorded. Both transient and maintained discharge patterns were found.

The boundaries and extent of the receptive fields were found to vary with light and dark adaptation. With high background illumination the receptive fields tended to shrink, while they tended to expand during dark adaptation. He also found that different regions within a single receptive field tended to interact: 'off'-areas tended to suppress the discharges from 'on'-areas and vice versa. In fact, all degrees of mutual modifications were obtained when different zones within the receptive field were activated simultaneously by the two test lights.

Furthermore, Kuffler found that the ratio of regions dominated by 'on' or 'off' differed in *different* receptive fields.

To explain his results, Kuffler suggested that specific small areas within a receptive field of a ganglion cell gave rise to predominantly inhibitory or excitatory impulses and that the discharge pattern of larger areas of the field depended on the summed effect of the pathways converging on the given ganglion cell.

The important question of whether the receptive field organization of a ganglion cell was the same for the rod and cone receptor systems was pursued by Barlow, Fitzhugh and Kuffler (1957). In the light-adapted state, they found, in accord with Kuffler (1953), the receptive field of ganglion cells of the cat retina to be arranged so that the central and peripheral regions of the field were mutually antagonistic, evoking electrical potentials of opposite sign regardless of whether the ganglion cell explored was an 'on'- or 'off'-centre unit. In the dark-adapted state, on the other hand, they did not find this antagonistic interaction, suggesting that the receptive field organization of the rod and cone systems, in fact, was based on quite different principles.

Further investigation, however, revealed that the mutually antagonistic interaction between the central and peripheral parts of the receptive field could be obtained under conditions where only cones and only rods were test stimulated. Hence, it was concluded that dark adaptation, not a change in the receptor system, reduced the antagonistic interactions of the receptive field.

To explain the lateral inhibition found, the authors pointed to several possibilities: horizontal, amacrine or bipolar cells could all be responsible.

They also suggested that lateral inhibition could play a role in the simultaneous contrast effects observed psychophysically and also explain the well-known psychophysical fact stressed by Lythgoe (1940, p. 40) that summation of the light stimulus was more marked in the dark- than the light-adapted state. In opposition to Lythgoe's explanation, however, they suggested, based on their own results, that less interaction existed in the dark-adapted state, and that the increase of the summation effect obtained when the eye became dark adapted was due to a reduction of lateral inhibition, not an increase in lateral summation.

8 The duplicity theory of R. Granit

The spikes recorded by Hartline and Kuffler with the microelectrode technique represented end products in a series of consecutive events in the retina, starting with absorption of photons. To gain information about these extremely complex events that preceded the discharges of the optic nerve fibres, the research workers had to rely on the measurements of the electroretinogram (ERG). Indeed, it was generally held that mechanisms underlying the ERG response directly determined the impulse pattern of the optic nerve.

The ERG technique was first employed in 1865 by Frithiof Holmgren, a Swedish physiologist. He applied a pair of electrodes to an eye and found that the galvanometer connected to the electrodes gave a marked deflection both when the eye was illuminated and when the light was turned off. (For a description of the development of this technique, see introduction section of Granit, 1963.)

8.1 SUPPORTING EVIDENCE FOR THE DUPLICITY THEORY FROM THE ERG TECHNIQUE

A very extensive review of the research literature on ERG was made by Granit (1947). Presuming that the ERG response represented an average reaction, reflecting the processes of activated photoreceptors, the evidence reviewed was found to support the duplicity theory, suggesting that there were two quite different ERG response patterns of the retina, the so-called E- and I-ERG responses – the former characteristic of rod-dominant and the latter of cone-dominant retinas.

The hypothesis that the ERG response of rod and cone retinas differed was based on evidence obtained by measuring the ERG under conditions where the relative contribution of the two receptor types

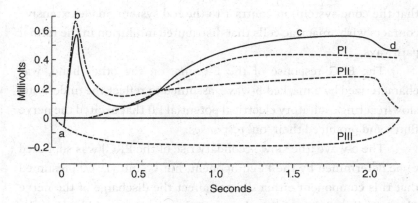

Fig. 8.1 A typical ERG curve as obtained by Granit (1938) with the multi-phasic fluctuation of potential; the characteristic a-, b-, c- and d-waves. These electrical changes have been analyzed by Granit into three components, PI, PII and PIII, as shown in the figure.

was varied, for example, by light- and dark-adapting the eye, by using retinas of different species where the relative number of rods and cones varied, and by using blue and deep red test lights. The most convincing evidence in favour of the hypothesis was obtained under conditions where the adaptation level of the eye changed. Thus, during long-term dark adaptation, for example, the ERG of a mixed rod-cone retina underwent both a Purkinje shift (the maximum spectral response changed from about 560 nm to about 500 nm) and a change from the I- to the E-ERG response.

The ERG of an E-retina containing both rods and cones is illustrated schematically in Fig. 8.1 where both the different waveforms (a, b, c and d) and the presumed underlying components (PI, PII and PIII) are shown. All these underlying components were found to be present in both types of retina, but to different degrees.

The ERG of the I-retina was characterized by marked a- and d-waves, assumed to be determined by the underlying PIII component, representing a rapidly reacting negative electrical potential. To account for this characteristic of the I-retina, Granit (1947) assumed that the cone system, in contrast to the rod system, made extensive contacts with amacrine cells that distributed inhibition in the retinal pathways.

The ERG response of the E-retina, on the other hand, was characterized by a marked b-wave, assumed to reflect the underlying slow-reacting excitatory electrical potential PII that excited the nerve fibres and produced their 'on' responses.

The c-wave (the slow secondary rise of the ERG) was supposed to be determined by the PI component, but Granit (1947) presumed that this component either did not affect the discharge of the nerve fibres at all or did so indirectly by altering the threshold level of the discharge.

Granit found further support of his explanation of the E- and I-retinas when he measured the change in the ERG response with light adaptation both in an E-retina containing rods and cones and in a pure I-retina containing only cones. Thus, while the E-retina showed a decrease in the b-wave (indicating a reduction of the excitatory PII underlying component) and a relative increase in the a- and d-waves (indicating a relative increase of the inhibitory PIII component), the pure I-retina showed no appreciable change in the form of its ERG.

He obtained another supporting finding with important theoretical implications under conditions where the light stimulus was flickering. In the E-retina the flickering light stimulus produced a sequence of b-waves (b-b-b-b-b), while the I-retina elicited alternating a- and b-waves (a-b-a-b-a-b). Also, the I-retina was able to follow a much higher flicker rate than the E-retina, presumably due to the rapidly reacting inhibitory PIII component that dominated the I-retina response. Accordingly, while the pure E-retina, containing no cones, would tend to elicit simple, relatively slow 'on'-responses in the nerve fibres, the I-retina would be able to produce complex, rapidly changing 'on-off' discharges.

Granit (1947) presumed that this characteristic of the I-retina gave extreme efficiency in transforming a visual field into frequency codes that could carry information about the physical world to the brain. Similarly, since PIII tended to increase relative to PII and also to react faster when the retina became light adapted, Granit held, in accordance with Lythgoe (1940), that light adaptation of a mixed rod-cone retina transformed it from a rod to a cone system, resetting the retinal instrument from slow to fast, and from integration to differentiation (see Granit, 1963, pp. 145–146).

Although the ERG measurement provided important information about the frequency pattern of the optic nerve fibres, Granit pointed out that the ERG was an average electrical response reflecting various electrical events in the retina, and that there was no simple relationship between the ERG measurements and the frequency of discharge of the optic nerve. Indeed, Granit found that the c-wave, produced by the PI component of the ERG, did not have any direct relationship to the impulse pattern of the optic nerve, and that the PIII component was chiefly concerned with inhibition of the optic nerve impulses. Measuring the impulse pattern in single fibres, as Hartline had done, might therefore provide a much better foundation when it came to the interpretation of psychophysical facts. Granit, inspired by this view, conducted a series of studies on various animal species to correlate variation in light stimulus and impulse pattern in single optic nerve fibres.

8.2 THE DOMINATOR-MODULATOR THEORY

The microelectrode technique employed was developed in the late 1930s by Granit and Svaetichin. It provided a supplement to Hartline's micro-dissection technique and had the important advantage that it could be applied to warm-blooded as easily as to cold-blooded species (see Granit, 1963, pp. 92–95). The cornea, lens and vitreous body were removed and the microelectrode applied to the inner surface of the retina with the aid of a micromanipulator. Spikes could then be recorded from what Granit assumed to be single or well-synchronized fibres. This assumption was based on the response characteristics recorded, such as the 'all-or-none' law, simplicity of record and duration of spikes.

By plotting the reciprocal of equal quantum intensity necessary to produce a threshold response against wavelength, Granit obtained so-called dominator and modulator curves. Two fundamentally different dominator curves were discovered in the mixed rod-cone retina: (1) a scotopic curve obtained under dark-adapted conditions with a maximum sensitivity at about 500 nm closely corresponding to the spectral curve of rhodopsin, and (2) a photopic dominator curve obtained under light-adapted conditions with a maximum sensitivity at about 560 nm. Thus, the change from the scotopic to the photopic curves represented a Purkinje shift – a shift from rod to cone activity. Accordingly, Granit found no photopic dominator curve in the rod retinas of the rat and guinea pig where, apparently, cone mechanisms of any significance were lacking.

8.2.1. The trichromatic colour theory challenged

Granit suggested that both the scotopic and photopic dominators served pure colourless 'white' sensation, since their spectral sensitivity curves were broad and, therefore, could not offer the central mechanism any adequate cue for colour discrimination. Accordingly, in sharp contrast to the Young-Helmholtz colour theory, he suggested that information about hue could only be conveyed by narrow spectral-sensitivity curves confined to widely separated spectral regions. In agreement with this view, he found, in addition to the dominator curves, numerous relatively light-resistant, narrow spectral modulator curves across the visible spectrum. Hence, these modulators appeared to be well suited for mediating wavelength information.

Nevertheless, although Granit stressed that the modulator curves were too narrow to be regarded as the trichromatic units of the Young-Helmholtz colour theory, he held that his results confirmed the essential truth of Thomas Young's generalizations, since the modulator curves were obtained in three different regions of the spectrum (440–470 nm, 520–540 nm and 580–610 nm).

Granit found a more severe challenge confronting the trichromatic theory in the observation that brightness and chromatic colour sensations may operate independently of each other. Thus, as already pointed out by Tschermak (1902, 1929) and von Kries (1911), a chromatic sensation may change to an achromatic sensation when, for example, size or intensity of a test field is reduced. This observation, of course, clearly opposed the Young-Helmholtz colour theory, but could easily be explained by Granit's dominator-modulator theory on his assumptions that (1) modulators (mediators of hue sensation) and dominators (mediators of achromatic sensation only) were activated by different receptor units, and (2) dominators were much more numerous than modulators. (Granit, though, admitted that Hering's colour theory, with its 'white-black' independent colour mechanism, could also explain the apparent independence of achromatic and chromatic sensations in a straightforward manner.)

Granit's dominator-modulator theory also offered a quite new explanation of various forms of colour-blindness. Thus, Granit (1947), in opposition to the trichromatic colour theory, suggested that deficiency of colour vision may depend on the absence of modulator mechanisms or their sensitivity reduction, changes in the relative number of modulators and dominators, and changes in dominator mechanisms. Rod monochromacy, for example, could be explained simply on the assumption that the photopic dominator and all the modulators were missing.

8.3 SCHULTZE'S DUPLICITY THEORY CHALLENGED

Interestingly, in mixed rod-cone retinas the photopic dominator response obtained from single units was often found to change to a scotopic dominator response during dark adaptation. This evidence strongly indicated that both rods and cones could activate the same nerve fibre, and that a given fibre, therefore, could carry messages from both rods and cones as had previously been suggested by Polyak (1941). In the dark-adapted state the response would be determined by the properties of rhodopsin, and the scotopic sensitivity curve would be obtained, while in photopic vision the sensitivity curve would depend on the integrative response of a number of different types of cone receptors connected to the fibre under investigation.

An even more interesting finding was that a dominator (assumed to mediate achromatic sensation) and a modulator (assumed to mediate hue sensation) could be obtained from the same fibre. To solve this problem, Granit suggested that the quality of the dominator and modulator responses was served by specialized fibre response patterns. Thus, he suggested that single nerve fibres were able to convey qualitatively different messages to the brain, a possibility also acknowledged by Helmholtz (1867) and Polyak (1941). In order to account for this violation of Helmholtz's (1896) specific fibre-energy doctrine (i.e. that a given nerve fibre transmitted a certain 'quality' independently of the nature of the stimulus), Granit (1947, 1955) presumed that excitatory and inhibitory impulses in the retina may interact and, thereby, produce a variety of frequency patterns in single nerve fibres conveying different kinds of information. Indeed, he suggested that different kinds of information could be transmitted *simultaneously* in the same fibre (see Granit, 1955, pp. 287–291). Such a powerful frequency-coding mechanism would, of course, allow rods and cones to function independently of each other in common pathways when both the receptor systems were simultaneously active.

Yet, in opposition to this view, Granit (1947) held that cone and rod activities tended to suppress each other when activated simultaneously. Clearly, one would expect the fast reacting negative electrical potential of the cones (PIII), chiefly concerned with inhibition, to suppress rod activity, but Granit also found strong evidence that the slow reacting positive electrical potential of the rods (PII) may inhibit cone activity. For instance, he showed that the fast cone component of the ERG obtained under photopic conditions tended to disappear after the eye had become completely dark adapted (see Granit, 1938, pp. 64–66, 1963, pp. 146–147).

The assumption of the orthodox duplicity theory of Schultze (1866) that rods only mediate achromatic vision was also challenged by Granit's finding of both blue and green modulators in the guinea pig retina presumed to be without cones. (Today, it is known that the guinea pig retina contains about 10% cones; see Yin *et al.*, 2006.)

Furthermore, Granit found a modulator curve with maximum sensitivity at about 500 nm that differed from the others in two respects. It was less resistant to light adaptation and was missing from pure cone retinas.

To explain these findings Granit (1947) suggested that, from a phylogenetic point of view, the modulators represented more primitive mechanisms than the photopic dominator mechanisms. They were assumed to be nature's first attempt, sometimes even serving rods, to organize wavelength discrimination, while the photopic dominator mechanisms were thought to be developed later and to be the result of an integration of several modulators. Furthermore, he suggested that cone-like rods existed that were relatively resistant to light adaptation, had high thresholds and contained rhodopsin which was chemically slightly different from the usual form found in ordinary dark-adapting rods. These cone-like rods were assumed to remain active after light adaptation and to be capable of mediating responses in the photopic state. Also, in agreement with Lythgoe (1940), Granit suggested that illumination of rhodopsin might be an essential factor in creating photopigments like those in cones.

9 Contributions of E. N. Willmer, P. Saugstad & A. Saugstad, and I. Lie

The new discoveries of Polyak, Hartline, Kuffler and Granit clearly indicated that the old orthodox formulation of the duplicity theory had serious flaws. In particular, the seminal discovery of Polyak and Granit that rods shared neural pathways with cones appeared to contradict the basic assumption of the theory that rods and cones functioned independently of each other. Obviously, the time was ripe for a reformulation of the theory to make its statements consistent with the new discoveries. In addition to the reformulations proposed by Polyak and Granit (see above), important changes to the theory were made both by Willmer (1946, 1961), Saugstad and Saugstad (1959) and Lie (1963).

Willmer's reformulation represented a quite new version of the duplicity theory. Indeed, he held that the rods under photopic conditions played an important role in trichromatic colour vision.

Saugstad and Saugstad called for a more moderate revision of the theory. They held that its statements should be reformulated making the meaning more explicit. Also, they pointed to well-founded evidence against the theory and concluded that its statements should be qualified by the development of a more comprehensive theory, taking into account the structure and function of the nervous system.

The contributions of Willmer and Saugstad and Saugstad were primarily theoretical. Lie, on the other hand, made a thorough empirical, psychophysical investigation focused on rod-cone interactions in colour vision under mesopic test conditions. In opposition to the orthodox conception of the duplicity theory, he interpreted his results to mean that rod and cone activities in the retina antagonized each other over a long transitional mesopic-intensity interval.

The hypotheses of Polyak, Granit, Willmer, Saugstad and Saugstad and Lie represented a radical break with the previous, long-held assumptions of separation and independence between the rod and cone functions. Together they made a strong case for the idea of rod-cone interactions at the retinal level.

9.1 THE DUPLICITY THEORY OF WILLMER

The new version of the duplicity theory put forward by Willmer (1946) was intended to stimulate research and promote new experimental investigations. Yet, he admitted that his theory was both speculative, provocative and not able to account for all important colour phenomena.

As a basic premise, he held that there were four primary mechanisms in the human retina. This had been proved by previous research work. Thus, Maxwell (1855, 1860) had shown that the retinal colour response to spectral lights involved a triplex mechanism, and König (1894) had shown that a separate rod receptor mechanism functioned in scotopic vision. Also, König and Dieterici (1893), in a very comprehensive study on colour vision and spectral sensitivity in monochromats, dichromats, and normal and anomalous trichromats, had demonstrated that a minimum of four primary processes (Grundempfindungen) were needed to explain their results.

Yet, there was no agreement on the anatomical substrate of the four primary mechanisms. Indeed, Schultze (1866) and Polyak (1941) had found that only two different types of receptor, rods and cones, could be differentiated in the human retina by histological examination. Hence, the question naturally arose of how these two receptor types could account for the four primary mechanisms.

9.1.1 *Colour vision explained by two types of rod and one type of cone*

Willmer (1946) attempted to solve this problem by suggesting that the human retina contained two different types of rod and one type of cone, and that two of the four primary mechanisms were served by rods interacting with cones. Thus he presumed that:

1. The primary 'red' mechanism was subserved by signals from cones with maximum sensitivity at about 590 nm transmitted through Polyak's midget bipolar cells.
2. The primary 'green' mechanism was subserved by impulses originating in the 'red' (590 nm) cones and in so-called 'day rods'. These impulses were combined and transmitted through Polyak's flat bipolar cells and determined a spectral sensitivity curve with maximum sensitivity at about 535 nm. The 'day-rods' differed from the ordinary dark-adapting rods in that they did not have the ability to accumulate rhodopsin in any measurable quantity. Hence, they could not increase their sensitivity during the second phase of long-term dark adaptation.
3. The primary 'blue' mechanism was subserved by impulses from the dark-adapting rods being partially inhibited by the 'red' (590 nm) cones. Due to this inhibition the spectral sensitivity of the rods was assumed to change from that of rhodopsin (maximum sensitivity at about 500 nm) to that of the primary 'blue' colour mechanism (maximum sensitivity at about 450 nm) as test conditions changed from scotopic to photopic. Thus, at variance with König's (1894) assumption that the bleaching product of rhodopsin, 'visual yellow', was responsible for the primary 'blue' mechanism, Willmer presumed that it was an effect of cone-rod interaction.
4. Finally, the fourth mechanism was subserved by signals from the ordinary dark-adapting rods.

As can be seen, the theory introduced by Willmer (1946) involved only one type of cone and two types of rod receptor, while the duplicity theory of von Kries (1911) operated with one rod receptor type and three types of cone. Also, in sharp contrast to the basic assumption of the duplicity theory that rods and cones functioned independently of each other, Willmer (1946) made rod-cone interaction a prerequisite for trichromatic colour vision. Thus, both the 'blue' and 'green' primaries were served by rods interacting with cones. Obviously, these radical, new ideas of rod-cone interaction needed solid underpinning in order to gain general acceptance.

9.1.2 Evidence supporting Willmer's duplicity theory

Willmer (1946) pointed to three different experimental findings in support of the view that ordinary dark-adapting rods under photopic condition constituted the primary 'blue' receptor mechanism:

1. Experiments had shown the rod-free fovea to be tritanopic, or 'blue-blind', i.e. unable to discriminate between wavelengths in the short-wave region of the spectrum (König, 1894; Willmer, 1946).
2. The tritanopic state was also found to emerge during dark adaptation in the extrafovea when the test condition changed from *photopic* to *mesopic*, i.e. when the cone inhibition of the ordinary, dark-adapting rod receptors was assumed to decrease.
3. Finally, Willmer pointed to the finding of Granit that the rod-retina of the guinea pig showed clear evidence of a relative increase in sensitivity to the blue part of the spectrum when the eye became light adapted.

Moreover, Willmer could present a plausible case in evolutionary terms. His reasoning ran as follows: in the course of the evolutionary development, rods had gained their remarkable sensitivity by increasing their content of rhodopsin and so had become useful under conditions of low illumination. They had also become inordinately sensitive under daylight conditions causing dazzling at high intensity levels – as clearly evidenced by the visual behaviour of rod monochromats. If, then, the less sensitive cones had developed an inhibitory mechanism that counteracted the extreme increase in rod sensitivity and at the same time had created the photopic 'blue' primary, this would surely have been a phylogenetic development of great survival value.

He also found evidence for the inhibitory cone mechanisms in the results obtained by Granit. Thus, by examining the waveform of the electroretinogram (ERG) of the retina, Granit had provided evidence that the mixed rod-cone retina was more inhibited in the light-adapted than in the dark-adapted eye, and that in the light-adapted eye the mixed rod-cone retina was more inhibited than the pure rod retina.

Finally, in support of his basic assumption that the retina contained more than one type of rod, Willmer pointed to the observation of Kühne that rods in the extreme periphery of the human retina and also in a region close to the central fovea were devoid of rhodopsin (Kühne, 1879, see pp. 263–264). He also mentioned the observation of Boll (1878) that the frog retina contained two different rod receptor types each with its own photopigment.

9.1.3 Reformulation of Willmer's duplicity theory

In 1961, Willmer reformulated his theory. He still maintained the hypothesis that the ordinary dark-adapting rods by being inhibited by cones constituted the 'blue' receptor mechanism in photopic vision, but abandoned his hypothesis of 'day-rods', since the results of Rushton (1957) strongly indicated that the retina contained at least two different types of cone photopigments. Thus, by measuring the capacity of different spectral lights to bleach photopigments in the human fovea, Rushton obtained evidence of two photo-labile cone pigments with spectral sensitivities similar to Stiles's 'red' and 'green' primaries. Willmer (1961), in accord with this finding, presumed that the retina, in addition to the primary 'blue' rod mechanism, contained a primary 'red' and a primary 'green' cone-based mechanism.

Another important improvement of the theory was his determination of the spectral sensitivity functions of these two primary cone receptor mechanisms. For this purpose he exploited an ingenious technique. Taking advantage of the finding that the central fovea lacked the primary 'blue' mechanism, he could single out and measure the spectral sensitivity of the 'red' and 'green' primaries by examining, respectively, deutranope (green-blind) and protanope (red-blind) subjects, since they all became monochromatic when test stimulated in the central 'blue-blind' fovea (the fovea of deutranope and protanope being subserved, respectively, only by the 'red' and 'green' primary mechanism).

The procedure employed to obtain the spectral sensitivity of the 'blue' primary mechanism, on the other hand, was much more complicated and expressed by the mathematical equation:

$$B = R - K \left(C - C_0 \right)$$

where B is the effective response from rods that generates the spectral sensitivity of the 'blue' primary, R and C the immediate responses from, respectively, rods and cones, C_0 the threshold response at which the cones begin to inhibit the rods, and K a constant equal to 1.75.

It should be noted that the primary 'blue' mechanism was assumed to consist of two underlying mechanisms. Thus, presuming that the primary 'red' and 'green' cone receptor systems may inhibit the rod receptor system somewhat differently, Willmer (1961) derived two 'blue' mechanisms with spectral sensitivities that closely matched the 'blue' π_1 and π_3 mechanisms obtained by Stiles with his well-known two-colour threshold technique (see Stiles, 1978).

Having determined the spectral sensitivities of four colour mechanisms operating in photopic vision, Willmer (1961) attempted to increase the explanatory power of his theory by incorporating new assumptions to account for the opponent characteristics of colour vision that Hering (1878) had called attention to. Thus, the 'red' and 'green' cone receptors were assumed to activate 'red-green' opponent cells where the 'red' cones generated a red colour by increasing the positive potential of the cells, while the 'green' cones generated a blue-green colour by increasing the negative potential of the cells.

The 'red' and 'green' cones were also assumed to activate 'yellow-blue' opponent cells, generating a yellow colour by increasing the positive potential of the cells, while the photopic rod activity was assumed to generate a bluish (indigo) colour by increasing the negative potential of these cells.

9.1.4 *Evidence supporting rods as 'blue' primaries*

The formula $B = R - K \left(C - C_0 \right)$ represented the most basic and original assumption of the second version of Willmer's (1961) theory, and he made a thorough attempt to underpin it. Firstly, he presented a long list of circumstantial evidence where he showed the characteristics of the 'blue' mechanism to differ from the 'red' and 'green' mechanisms and that some of the properties of the primary 'blue' mechanism had features in common with the ordinary dark-adapting rods. Thus, for example, he noted that while deuteranopia and protanopia were inherited as sex-linked allelomorphs, tritanopia (blue-blindness) was inherited quite separately as an autosomal recessive condition. Thus, the genes for the development of the structures responsible for the 'blue' mechanism, like those of the rod mechanism, were carried on a different chromosome from the genes for the 'red-green' complex. He also noted that the Weber fractions (that is, the ratio of a just detectable increase in intensity to the intensity of the stimulus) measured for the 'blue' and the rod mechanisms were strikingly similar and so were their receptive field sizes.

More substantial evidence was found in the results of Trezona (1960) that a positive, blue afterimage observed in darkness after a strong 'white' bleach may be readily obtained just outside the fovea where rods are activated, but not in the rod-free central fovea (it should be noted that this positive, blue afterimage appears akin to the so-called positive, complementary Purkinje afterimage, discussed by von Kries, 1929). Willmer (1961) also pointed to the fact that blue, violet and purple colours in many instances were associated with twilight vision.

Yet, Willmer's most convincing evidence appears to be some remarkable results he obtained in an experiment on simultaneous contrast, where he found that an inducing field of long wavelength, assumed to activate mostly cones, could generate a blue colour in a test field assumed to activate only rods. The same blue colour was observed independently of both the test wavelength (varied between 400 and 580 nm) and the inducing wavelength (varied between 580 and 700 nm) (see Willmer, 1950).

9.1.5 Evidence opposing rods as 'blue' primaries
Finally, in order to complete his argument, Willmer (1961) scrutinized objecctions that could be raised against his basic assumption that rods may represent the primary 'blue' mechanism under photopic conditions:

1. Rods in photopic vision would be saturated over a large part of the spectrum from violet to yellow and, hence, be unable to discriminate between wavelengths in this region.
2. A match between two colour fields made under photopic conditions would break down under scotopic conditions (the Purkinje phenomenon).
3. The Stiles-Crawford directional effect, found in the blue region of the spectrum, was absent under scotopic conditions.
4. The spectral sensitivity curve for rhodopsin could not be obtained by any linear transformation of the colour-mixture curves.

Willmer's (1961) inquiry led him to conclude that each of the objections could be surmounted, since they all presumed that the dark-adapting rods constituted the primary 'blue' receptor mechanism, while his theory implied that the dark-adapting rod activity was drastically modified at photopic intensity levels by cone activity.

Although Willmer's ingenious but speculative colour theory adequately explained many of the basic facts of colour vision, its distinguishing mark, that the ordinary dark-adapting rods under photopic conditions represented the primary 'blue' receptor mechanism, was shown to be wrong only a few years after the second version of his theory had been published. In 1964, it was conclusively demonstrated that the retina actually contained three types of cone as had been generally presumed (see Marks *et al.*, 1964; Brown & Wald, 1964). By measuring the absorption spectra of single parafoveal receptors from the primate retina, these researchers found three types of cone each with its own photopigment. The maximum absorptions of the pigments were found in the violet, yellow-green and green-yellow parts of the spectrum. Furthermore, Wald (1964, 1967), using a limiting case of the two-colour threshold technique of Stiles, presented strong evidence for three kinds of cone within the rod-free fovea of the human retina. From now on it became universally accepted that the sensation of hue in photopic vision in normal trichromats was mediated by three types of cone.

In the early 1900s most of the research workers presumed that the desaturation effect of rod activity under mesopic test conditions was due to some unknown brain processes or was of a psychic nature.

with no counterpart in physiology. (See Helmholtz's, 1911, vol. III, pp. 24–29, discussion on how inductive conclusions, unconsciously formed, may influence perception.) Willmer's (1946) theory represented a radical break with these ideas. Thus, he made rod-cone interaction at the retinal level a central part of his theory. This strong emphasis on rod-cone interaction in the nervous system was also advanced by Saugstad and Saugstad (1959). The change in focus is clearly revealed when von Kries's (1929) classical review of the duplicity theory is compared with the evaluation of the theory given by Saugstad and Saugstad (1959) 30 years later. While Saugstad and Saugstad made the concept of rod-cone interaction in the retina their central point of discussion, the concept of rod-cone interaction was barely mentioned by von Kries.

9.2 SAUGSTAD AND SAUGSTAD: EVALUATION OF SCHULTZE'S DUPLICITY THEORY

The paper of Saugstad and Saugstad (1959) represents a painstaking attempt to review and evaluate all major evidence for and against the duplicity theory. Indeed, it may be considered the most thorough evaluation of the empirical basis of the theory ever made and will, therefore, be dealt with in some detail. Previous reviews had been published by Hecht (1937) and Lythgoe (1940).

9.2.1 Reformulation of Schultze's duplicity theory

Saugstad and Saugstad (1959) considered Schultze's (1866) formulation of the theory vague and inexplicit. They therefore found it necessary, before evaluating the theory, to reformulate its basic assumptions to make the implicit meaning clearer.

Firstly, they interpreted Schultze's (1866) theory to mean that rods did not, *under any condition*, mediate chromatic vision. This reformulation, of course, highlighted the controversy between the orthodox duplicity theory and the suggestions of König (1894) and Willmer (1946) that rods, under certain conditions, generated a blue colour sensation.

Secondly, they interpreted the duplicity theory to mean that each of the two receptor types functioned identically in different species, and that the retina did not contain any other visual receptor type.

Finally, they interpreted the theory to mean that rods and cones formed two completely separated visual systems without any interaction and that there, consequently, was *no* common intensity interval where the two receptor types functioned together. This interpretation of the duplicity theory was not intended by Schultze (1866), who had suggested that there was a mesopic intensity range where both receptor types were activated producing a combined effect. Yet, from Schultze's suggestion, several important, specific questions naturally arise:

1. What is the extent of the overlapping mesopic intensity interval?
2. What is the mechanism underlying the rod-cone interaction?
3. Do the answers found for one visual function apply to all?

The somewhat extreme interpretation of the duplicity theory by Saugstad and Saugstad (1959) may thus be seen as an attempt to highlight these basic questions not addressed by Schultze (1866).

Saugstad and Saugstad (1959) also drew attention to yet another serious weakness inherent in Schultze's (1866) theory: it attributed the duplex functioning of the visual system to differences between the rod and cone *receptors*. In view of Polyak's (1941) investigation of the connections of the various types of neural cells in the retina they found, in accord with Willmer (1946), this basic assumption to be quite untenable. Indeed, the thorough histological study of Polyak (1941) had revealed that rods and cones had common pathways. Obviously, these common pathways provided strong support for the assumption that the two receptor systems interacted even as early as at the retinal level, and that interaction might be found under a variety of conditions. Yet, Saugstad and Saugstad (1959) did not preclude the possibility that rods and cones might operate within different intensity intervals through mechanisms of neural inhibition and facilitation.

On the basis of their reformulation, Saugstad and Saugstad (1959) then made a thorough and systematic evaluation of the empirical basis of the duplicity theory. They concluded that although there was ample and well-founded evidence in support of a duality of function between the two basically different types of receptor, there was also ample, if not equally well-founded, evidence pointing to a need for a revision and elaboration of the theory. In particular, they stressed the need for its statements to be qualified by being developed into a more comprehensive theory by including known structures and functions of the nervous substrate of the visual system.

9.2.2 Evidence in support of Schultze's duplicity theory

In support of the duplicity theory they presented the following evidence:

1. The spectral sensitivity curves obtained under photopic and scotopic conditions had been found to differ markedly with maximum sensitivity at about 560 nm and 510 nm, respectively.
2. Dark adaptation curves obtained by measuring the change in absolute threshold or the critical frequency of a flickering light (i.e. the fusion frequency) displayed one branch under photopic test conditions and another, quite different one, under scotopic test conditions.
3. The Purkinje shift obtained within the central fovea had been found to be much smaller than that obtained in the extrafoveal regions.
4. Studies of night blind and complete colour-blind subjects indicated that one of the two receptor types may be left intact while the other is impaired.
5. The retinal directional sensitivity, i.e. the change in sensitivity with a change of incident light angle, was mainly connected to cones.
6. Two different photochemical substances had been found; the rod photopigment rhodopsin that determined the scotopic-luminosity curve and the cone photopigment iodopsin that determined the photopic-luminosity curve (Wald, 1937b).
7. Pure cone and pure rod retinas had been found only in diurnal and in nocturnal species, respectively.

9.2.3 *Evidence against Schultze's duplicity theory*

Despite the strong supporting evidence that the retina contained two different types of photoreceptor subserving different functions, Saugstad and Saugstad (1959) also presented a long list of carefully conducted studies that clearly showed that the duplicity theory needed revision and elaboration. Their main concern was the question of rod-cone interaction. On the basis of their interpretation of the theory, they predicted that there should be an abrupt change-over from rod to cone function as intensity increased from scotopic to photopic levels, or vice versa, irrespective of function measured. Opposed to this prediction, however, the available evidence suggested that, for several visual functions, rods and cones were activated simultaneously and produced a combined effect over a considerable range of intensities. A number of classical studies supported this conclusion.

Firstly, Walters and Wright (1943) had found that when the test intensity increased from scotopic to photopic levels, the change of the spectral sensitivity curve, measured psychophysically in the extrafovea, was gradual and continuous over a very wide intensity range and not abrupt as would be expected from the duplicity theory. Furthermore, they found that the spectral sensitivity curve obtained at the highest intensity level employed (more than 3 log units above absolute cone threshold) was not identical to that obtained at the fovea, but displaced toward the rod curve. These results, then, strongly suggested that rod and cone signals may function simultaneously and interact with regard to brightness.

The same interpretation could be applied to the results obtained by Blanchard (1918) on light adaptation. He found that the incremental-threshold curve of an extrafoveal, white test light (i.e. the logarithm of the absolute threshold level of the test light plotted against the logarithm of the intensity of an adapting background light) yielded a continuous straight line instead of an abrupt change in the gradient where the transition from the rod to the cone system was expected to occur.

Similarly, a review on change in brightness discrimination with changes in background intensity showed no clear breaks in the extrafoveal curves. The results, therefore, were judged to indicate overlapping and interaction of the brightness functions of rods and cones.

Furthermore, evidence presented by Lythgoe (1940) strongly indicated that rod and cone impulses may also interact to determine the fusion frequency of a flickering light. Measuring the fusion frequency in the extrafoveal retina during dark adaptation whilst the illumination of the flickering light was kept constant, he found, in accord with the duplicity theory, that the fusion frequency fell or rose depending on whether the test illumination activated the photopic or scotopic mechanism, respectively. However, the results displayed no clear-cut change-over from fall to rise during the dark-adaptation period. Instead, they strongly indicated that cones determined the critical frequency measurements during the first part of the dark-adaptation curve, both receptor mechanisms during the middle part and only rods during the last part.

Saugstad and Saugstad (1959) also presented evidence that challenged the basic assumption of Schultze (1866) that rods mediated achromatic vision only. Thus, evidence in support of the assumption that rods may mediate colours of short wavelengths was found in the results obtained by Hecht, Haig and Chase (1936/1937). Measuring the dark-adaptation curve following moderate light adaptation, they showed that the change from coloured to colourless perception for a violet test light in the extrafoveal retina could be obtained below the cone plateau level.

Furthermore, Kohlrausch (1931) obtained dark-adaptation curves with only one branch in the extrafoveal retina despite the fact that colours could be observed at the threshold level during the first part of the curve. Saugstad and Saugstad (1959) interpreted this result to mean that either the form of the curves was due to interaction between rod and cone activities, or, presuming that the curves were determined by rods alone, that rods mediated the colour sensations observed.

Moreover, in a study by Shlaer, Smith and Chase (1941/1942), it was found that visual acuity was better in the parafovea than in the fovea for blue, but not for red light. Saugstad and Saugstad (1959) suggested that this better acuity performance for the extrafoveal blue colour could be explained either as a combined effect of rods and cones, or as an effect of rods mediating colours of short wavelengths.

Finally, in support of rods as mediators of colour vision, Saugstad and Saugstad (1959) pointed out that Granit (1947) had found modulator curves in the presumed all-rod retina of the guinea-pig. Yet, they held that this evidence was weakened by the uncertainty of the cell type involved in the recording and of the response pathway from receptor to the recording site. They held that there was no consensus as to whether or not the guinea-pig had an entirely cone-free retina.

Saugstad and Saugstad (1959) also made an evaluation of the two remaining assumptions of the duplicity theory: (1) that only the rod and cone receptors, no other visual receptor types, existed in the retina, and (2) that each of the two receptor types functioned in the same way in different species.

As regards assumption (1), they argued that its empirical foundation was weak. Thus, they pointed out that the status of the receptors of the central fovea had not been agreed on. The receptors looked like rods but functioned like cones. Indeed, they suggested that the foveal receptors might constitute a third variety of photoreceptor, since evidence indicated that both spectral sensitivity (Walters & Wright, 1943), sensitivity change during dark adaptation (Hecht *et al.*, 1935/1936) and retinal directional sensitivity (Stiles, 1939) for foveal and extrafoveal cones may differ markedly.

Also, the empirical basis of assumption (2) was found to be weak. Two opposing arguments were put forward: (1) The structure of both rods and cones may differ markedly for different species, and (2) flicker responses plotted as a function of intensity had been found to be strikingly similar for the rod retina of the gecko and the cone retina of the turtle (Croizier & Wolf, 1938/1939).

The systematic evaluation of the duplicity theory by Saugstad and Saugstad could leave little doubt that there was ample room for improvement and further development of the duplicity theory. In particular, they stressed the lack of knowledge with regard to rod-cone interaction under mesopic conditions. The available evidence strongly suggested that rod and cone impulses interacted and produced a combined effect under a variety of mesopic test conditions, but the essential characteristics of the interaction processes were still largely unknown.

9.3 IVAR LIE: INTERACTIONS BETWEEN ROD AND CONE FUNCTIONS AT MESOPIC INTENSITY

9.3.1 Psychophysical experiments

Only a few years later, however, the question of how rods and cones interact under mesopic conditions was successfully addressed by Lie (1963). In an extensive psychophysical, empirical investigation, using a Hecth & Schlaer adaptometer (Hecth & Schlaer, 1938) he provided conclusive evidence that the achromatic rod and the chromatic cone components may interact in a kind of colour-mixing process.

In his investigation, Lie took advantage of the generally accepted assumption that cones dark adapt much faster than rods. Thus, it had long been known that following substantial bleaches, cones reach their maximum sensitivity after a few minutes of dark adaptation, while the rods may need more than 40 minutes to approach their final level. Hence, the effect of rod activity upon cone functions may be measured at mesopic intensity levels after the cones have reached their dark-adapted state and the rods still increase their sensitivity.

Loeser (1904) appears to be the first to utilize this ideal method under adequately controlled conditions. In this study he investigated how rod signals affected cone-mediated colour sensation when they intruded during long-term dark adaptation. During the first phase of the dark adaptation period, he found the absolute and the specific-hue thresholds (i.e. the intensity levels where the subject first becomes

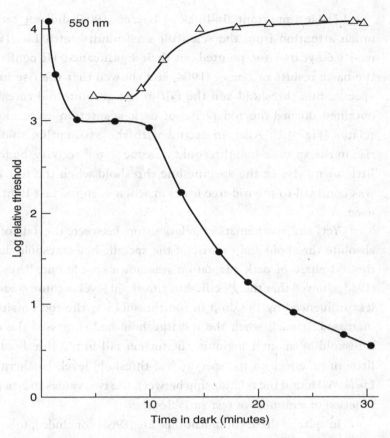

Fig. 9.1 Absolute (●) and specific-hue (Δ) thresholds of a 550 nm light (the absolute light and colour thresholds) measured at 7° extrafoveally during long-term dark adaptation. The test field was 1 × 1° exposed for 0.5 s.

aware of the light and colour of the test stimulus when the test intensity is increased from below) coincided for red, green and blue test lights. But thereafter, during the second phase of dark adaptation where only rods increased their sensitivity, the specific-hue threshold started to rise markedly for all the test colours. The rise was most pronounced for the blue and least for the red test colour. Presuming, in accord with Schultze and Parinaud, that rods mediated achromatic vision only, he explained the rise of the specific-hue threshold obtained simply by the increase in rod sensitivity.

These important findings of Loeser (1904) did not receive much attention from the scientific community until Lie (1963), nearly 60 years later, pointed out their significance. He confirmed the basic results of Loeser (1904) and showed that the rise in the specific-hue threshold and the fall in the absolute rod threshold obtained during the rod phase of dark adaptation were closely related (Fig. 9.1). Also, in accord with the assumption that the rise in the specific-hue threshold was due to rod activity, he found little or no rise in the specific-hue threshold when the test light was confined to the rod-free fovea or when deep-red test light was used.

Yet, the mathematical relationship between the fall of the absolute threshold and the rise of the specific-hue threshold during the rod phase of dark adaptation was not a simple one. Thus, Lie (1963) showed that the specific-hue threshold level became gradually less influenced by the drop in rod threshold as the rod sensitivity increased. Indeed, when the rod threshold had surpassed the cone threshold by about 1 log unit, the further fall in rod threshold had little or no effect on the specific hue-threshold level. Furthermore, Lie (1963) found the relationship between the two values to be a joint function of a number of test variables.

In spite of these complications, Lie (1963) concluded, in accord with the explanation given previously by Loeser (1904), that the rise of the specific-hue threshold was an effect of the increase of the rod activity.

In a separate experiment (Experiment 7), he compared the saturation and brightness of a green monochromatic test colour observed extrafoveally at intensities *above* the specific hue-threshold, during the cone-plateau period and in a dark-adapted state. He found that the test field observed in the dark-adapted state appeared more desaturated and bright. As the test intensity was increased, however, the difference in saturation and brightness decreased until, at about 1 log unit above the specific-hue threshold, he found saturation and brightness obtained during the cone-plateau period and in a dark-adapted state to be the same.

9.3.2 The colour-mixing hypothesis

Presuming that the sensitivity of cones stayed essentially constant, while the sensitivity of rods increased during the rod phase of dark adaptation, Lie (1963) explained his results (the rise of the specific-hue threshold during the rod phase of dark adaptation and the effects on saturation and brightness of dark adaptation obtained with the green test light, Experiment 7) by a colour-mixture hypothesis, where the cone and rod mechanisms contributed a chromatic and an achromatic component, respectively.

Presuming that the relative strength of the achromatic rod and the chromatic cone components varied with changes in the test conditions, he could also explain the changing relationship obtained between the fall in rod threshold and the rise in the specific-hue threshold when test conditions were varied.

9.3.3 An alternative explanatory model

Although Lie (1963) held that his simple colour-mixture hypothesis could account reasonably well for his results, he presented a more sophisticated, alternative explanatory model where he combined the colour-mixture hypothesis with a hypothesis of antagonistic retinal interaction between the rod and cone activities. In defence of this antagonistic interaction he argued that rod and cone impulses when activating the same nerve fibre simultaneously must be mutually exclusive since they mediate qualitatively different colour sensations.

With the alternative model he could explain change in colour with intensity observed in a dark-adapted state as follows:

When the eye is test stimulated with a monochromatic light between the absolute threshold and the cone-plateau level in a dark-adapted state, there is no antagonistic rod-cone interaction, since only the rod system is activated. The subject will therefore observe the test flash as achromatic.

When the test intensity reaches the cone-plateau level, fibres connected to both rods and cones will still be occupied with rod activity, since the cone impulses are inhibited by the stronger rod impulses. Nerve fibres connected solely to cones, on the other hand, become occupied with cone activity. However, the achromatic rod component in the colour-mixture process will be dominant so that the subject will not detect the small chromatic component involved.

As the test intensity increases further, the relative strength of the cone impulses gradually increases resulting in an increasing number of cone-occupied nerve fibres. Eventually, the subject will detect the so-called 'correct' hue of the test light. It should be noted that the change-over from rod to cone occupied nerve fibres was assumed to take place at different intensity levels for different fibres, depending on the sensitivity of the individual receptors and the number of cones relative to rods connected to each fibre.

When the test intensity increases above the specific-hue threshold level, the saturation of the test colour will increase as the number of cone-occupied nerve fibres increases.

At the highest intensity levels only fibres connected exclusively to rods will be occupied with rod activity. However, as indicated by his results obtained with the green test light (Experiment 7), the subjects would not be able to detect this small achromatic rod component in the colour-mixture process.

Although both his theoretical models could explain the data reasonably well, Lie (1963) pointed out that several important questions remained, and that his investigation should be expanded. In particular, he found it of interest to explore how the specific-hue threshold level changed with *light adaptation*. He predicted that if the mechanisms of light and dark adaptation were the same, the specific-hue threshold should be obtained at the same intensity level under mesopic test conditions when the absolute rod thresholds for dark and light adaptation under scotopic test conditions were the same. He held that this prediction should be subjected to an empirical test, but never engaged in such an investigation.

Lie (1963) also pointed out the lack of knowledge with regard to variation in the relative strength of the achromatic rod and chromatic cone component with test parameters.

Status of the duplicity theory in the mid 1960s and its further development

At the end of the mid-twentieth century period (1930–1966), spectrophotometric measurements of spectral absorption in single photoreceptors had conclusively demonstrated that the retina contained three different types of cone, each cone with only one photopigment, together with the rods that contained only rhodopsin. Hence, it had been proved that the speculative idea of König (1894) and Willmer (1946, 1961) that rods may function as the primary 'blue' receptor, Willmer's and Granit's ideas of 'day rods', Polyak's idea that the trichromacy of colour vision was based on three types of bipolar cell, and the dominator-modulator theory of Granit, were all wrong. Moreover, Lie (1963), in his important and comprehensive study, had found that rods under scotopic test conditions mediated achromatic colour sensations only, and that under mesopic test conditions they contributed an achromatic component, desaturating the chromatic cone component.

Apparently, with the exception of the idea of rod-cone interaction, the duplicity theory had become strikingly similar to the old, orthodox conceptions formulated by von Kries (1929).

10.1 ELABORATION AND REVISION OF THE TWO MOST BASIC ASSUMPTIONS OF SCHULTZE'S DUPLICITY THEORY

As can be seen, the developmental history of the duplicity theory in the 100 years between 1866 and 1966 may be characterized by complex and comprehensive theory constructions. Outstanding examples are the theories provided by Schultze (1866), Parinaud (1881, 1885), König (1894), von Kries (1929), G.E. Müller (1930), Polyak (1941), Granit (1947, 1955) and Willmer (1946, 1961).

Yet, important contributions to the development of the theory were also made by workers who focused on more limited aspects of the theory. The most important contributions were provided by research workers who made penetrating and thorough studies to uncover the underlying mechanisms of the most basic assumption of the duplicity theory, namely that rods alone operated in night vision and cones in day vision.

Schultze (1866) could not provide any explanation of this difference in rod and cone sensitivity, either in photochemical, anatomical or physiological terms. Following Boll's (1877) discovery of the bleaching and regeneration of rhodopsin, however, important insights into the sensitivity regulation mechanisms were provided by Kühne in the nineteenth century and by Hecht, Wald, Rushton, Barlow and Lamb in the twentieth century. In fact, their contributions may be seen as a mainthread in the developmental history of the duplicity theory.

Yet, contributions were also provided by research workers who presented evidence opposing Schultze's (1866) second major assumption that rods mediated achromatic vision only. Indeed, the evidence offered strongly suggested that the rod system was an important contributor to chromatic colour vision and that rod signals served achromatic vision only under scotopic conditions when the eye was in a dark-adapted and chromatically neutral state of adaptation. Thus, it was found that (1) rod signals of the primate retina were transferred to ganglion cells via cone pathways (Fig. 10.1) and fed both spectrally opponent and non-opponent colour cells (De Valois, 1965; Wiesel & Hubel, 1966; Daw et al., 1990; Lennie & Fairchild, 1994; Wässle et al., 1995); and (2) rod signals could give rise to all sorts of hue sensations when interacting with cone activity (Stabell, 1967a; Stabell & Stabell, 1973a, 1994; McCann & Benton, 1969; Stromeyer, 1974a, b; Buck, 1997). Obviously, a major reformulation of the duplicity theory was called for.

In the following part we will describe how our knowledge of the sensitivity regulation mechanisms of rods and cones and of the

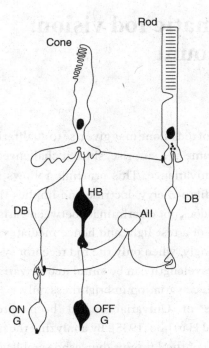

Fig. 10.1 Simplified illustration of how rod signals may affect cone activity in the primate retina. Signals from rods enter cone pathways via gap junctions between rod and cone receptors, and between AII (rod amacrine cells) and depolarizing cone-bipolar cells (illustrated by the DB cell in contact with the cone). A rod depolarizing bipolar cell (the DB cell in contact with the rod) is also shown. Moreover, signals from rods may affect hyperpolarizing cone-bipolar cells (illustrated by the HB cell) through conventional chemical synapses. ON G and OFF G represent on- and off-ganglion cells, respectively.

mechanism of chromatic rod vision developed, tracing the development back to its origin in the nineteenth century. We start with the development of the ideas of chromatic rod vision.

Part III Chromatic rod vision: a historical account

The finding that stimulation of rods alone may give rise to qualitatively different colour sensations came as a surprise, since it challenged the fundamental Principle of Univariance. This principle follows from Helmholtz's (1896) specific fibre-energy doctrine and implies that a given receptor or nerve fibre does not discriminate between variation in intensity and wavelength of a test light and hence mediates only one sensory quality. Accordingly, when only the rod receptor system is stimulated, variation in wavelength can be simulated by variation in intensity – they both produce variation in brightness only.

Indeed, the Principle of Univariance had been directly demonstrated by Graham and Hartline (1935). By analyzing the nerve impulses arising in the retina of the *Limulus* (horseshoe crab), where each photoreceptor is linked with a separate nerve fibre, they found that the variation in the response of the single fibres with wavelength could be simulated by suitably adjustment of the incident light energy. Thus, when the intensity was suitably adjusted, any test wavelength could be made to evoke the same frequency of impulses from a given receptor cell. Hence, it appeared that single retinal receptors alone had no power to discriminate between wavelength and intensity.

How, then, could the Principle of Univariance be reconciled with the new discovery that test stimulation of rods may give rise to all the principle hues of the spectrum? An answer to this question became apparent when it was discovered that the scotopic hues were due to rod-cone interactions. It followed that the Principle of Univariance and the specific fibre-energy doctrine of Helmholtz (1896) should only be applied to functionally independent receptor systems.

The origin of the idea that rods may give rise to chromatic sensations may be traced back to the hypothesis of Ebbinghaus (1893) that the photopigment of rods (rhodopsin) was the yellow-blue see-substance postulated by Hering (1878), and the suggestion of König (1894) that the rod receptors represented the primary 'blue' receptor system of photopic vision. Substantial evidence in favour of the idea was provided by von Kries and Nagel (1896) who found that twilight vision contained a tint of blue.

In order to identify more precisely this blue colour quality of rods, von Kries (1896) attempted to find the spectral light that did not change its hue when test intensity was reduced from photopic to scotopic levels, i.e. when the rod component increased. He used Nagel (a deutranope) as his subject and instructed him first to make a colour match at a photopic intensity level between a homogeneous spectral test light from the short-wave region of the spectrum (and hence with a relatively high potential scotopic value) and a mixture of spectrum red (670 nm) and violet (435 nm) lights (and hence with a relatively low potential scotopic value). Thereafter, the intensity of the test and comparison fields was reduced in the same proportion from the photopic level until the homogeneous light strongly activated the rod component. His results showed that the spectral light that did not change in colour quality with intensity reduction was situated between 480–485 nm, i.e. in the green-blue part of the spectrum.

Dreher (1912) made a somewhat similar investigation using two trichromats as subjects and confirmed the results of von Kries. G. E. Müller (1923), in his review on the colour quality of night vision, also concluded that, in addition to the dominant achromatic component, it entailed a tint of green-blue. He presumed that this green-blue colour was generated when light activated rhodopsin, but could not decide with certainty whether the rhodopsin molecules generating the green-blue colour were situated in the outer segment of rods or cones, although he thought it most likely that the green-blue colour had a rod origin.

It should be noted, however, that there was no general agreement as to the colour quality of night vision. Most subjects described night vision as achromatic. Even von Kries (1896, p. 87) found the word 'farblos' ('colourless') an appropriate description. Thus, in a footnote he remarked,

> Es wäre also vielleicht richtiger, nicht zu sagen, dass die Stäbchen farblose Empfindungen, sondern dass sie einen nur einsinnig veränderlichen Empfindungseffekt liefern. Da indessen der Stäbcheneffekt sich schwerlich in erheblichem Masse von der Farblosigkeit im gewöhnlichen Sinne unterscheidet, so schien es mir besser, den obigen, seine Bedeutung jedenfalls sehr viel anschaulicher kennzeichnenden Ausdruck beizubehalten.
>
> (Thus it might be more correct not to say that the rods give rise to colourless sensations, but that they give rise to one quality only. Yet, since the rod effect does not differ much from what is generally considered as achromatic sensation, it appears to me better to retain the above expression, which, at any rate, gives a far more elucidating characterization.)

The discrepancy between the reports of different subjects with regard to the colour quality of night vision could most easily be explained by individual differences. Yet, an alternative and more fruitful hypothesis was offered by Nagel (1911). He assumed that the colour quality of twilight vision, for *each* subject, may vary from colourless to blue. Thus, he wrote, 'Incidentally, it is quite conceivable that the light sensations that occur under the condition of pure twilight vision have a certain range of fluctuation as to their quality, varying from absolute colourlessness to a cyan-blue of no little saturation' (Nagel, 1911, p. 350). He assumed that this change in colour quality was due to some unknown adaptation mechanism.

The important hypothesis of Nagel (1911) that the colour quality of scotopic vision may vary with conditions of adaptation was also suggested by the results of a simultaneous contrast experiment performed by Willmer (1950). In this experiment he had found that the colour quality of a test field presented at an intensity level below the specific-hue threshold (but not necessarily below the absolute cone threshold) changed from achromatic to bluish when a chromatic long-wave inducing field was applied. Presupposing that the test field activated rods only, he assumed that the change from achromatic to blue resulted from interacting rod and cone activities, supporting his suggestion that the rods constituted the 'primary' blue receptor of photopic vision. Thus, he speculated that the blue colour observed in daylight was due to rod activity that escaped inhibition from cones (Willmer, 1961).

As we have seen, this speculation of Willmer was disproved by spectrophotometrical measurements that demonstrated the existence of 'blue' cone receptors. Yet, the more general presumption of Willmer, that rods and cones may interact to produce hue sensations, was supported by a preliminary study of Stabell and Stabell designed to determine the first appearance of rod activity following substantial bleaching. Thus, the subject should decide when the colour of the test field presented at a mesopic intensity level first changed during the long-term dark-adaptation period. On the basis of Lie's (1963) results, it was expected that the rod intrusion would be marked by a sudden desaturation change (Stabell, 1967b). Surprisingly, however, it was found that a test colour that appeared green during the cone-plateau period suddenly changed markedly towards blue-violet in addition to being desaturated. To ascertain that this blue-violet colour obtained was actually generated by rods, the test intensity was dimmed to a scotopic intensity level. The results obtained confirmed the suggestion, and hence revealed that rods could trigger both blue-violet and achromatic colours depending on the chromatic state of adaptation.

This finding raised the question of whether the mechanisms underlying achromatic colour in scotopic and photopic vision actually were analogous. The question was whether the achromatic aspect of rod vision could be accounted for by the suggestion that opponent chromatic colour processes activated by rod signals antagonized each other completely when the eye was stimulated at scotopic intensities in a chromatically neutral state of adaptation. If this suggestion was correct, one would expect that by selectively chromatic adaptation of the eye, it would be possible to obtain every principle hue of the spectrum when test stimulating at scotopic intensities.

12 Mechanisms of chromatic rod vision in scotopic illumination

12.1 ALL PRINCIPLE HUES MAY BE OBSERVED IN SCOTOPIC VISION

A test of the prediction was carried out by Stabell and Stabell (1965). The successive phases of the experiment were as follows: (1) Dark adaptation for 30 min. (2) Pre-stimulation extrafoveally for 30 s using one of several colour filters in front of the eye at an intensity 1 log unit above the specific-hue threshold measured for the filter used. (3) Dark adaptation for 30 s. (4) Test stimulation at scotopic intensity levels in the pre-stimulated area using a green monochromatic test light.

Pre-stimulation with a red colour filter produced a blue colour upon the scotopic test stimulation, a yellow pre-stimulation filter produced blue or blue-violet, a green filter, blue-violet or violet, while blue and blue-green filters did not produce any chromatic effect upon scotopic test stimulation.

The reason for the failure to produce red, yellow and green scotopic contrast colours soon became apparent in a follow-up study where it was found that by increasing the level of chromatic adaptation (i.e. increasing the time of pre-stimulation, reducing the time interval between pre- and test stimulation, and increasing the size of the pre- and test-fields) scotopic red, orange and green colours could be produced. Thus, pre-stimulation with a green-blue colour produced a red colour upon test stimulation at scotopic intensities, a blue colour produced orange, and a purple colour produced a blue-green colour. Furthermore, it was found that blue and green scotopic contrast colours could be produced by simultaneous contrast where the inducing field was illuminated by a deep-red light (see Stabell, 1967a).

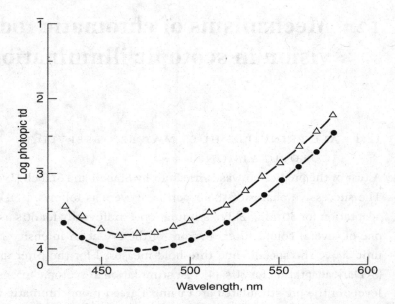

Fig. 12.1 Spectral threshold curves of scotopic contrast hues subsequent to pre-stimulation with 670 nm for 10 s at a retinal illumination of 3 photopic troland (Δ) together with absolute spectral threshold curve of rods measured in a completely dark-adapted eye (●). Both the test- and pre-stimulation fields were applied 6° temporally to the fovea. The size of the pre- and test- stimulation fields was 1 × 1° and the test flash was exposed for 0.5 s.

12.2 SCOTOPIC CONTRAST COLOURS ARE TRIGGERED BY ROD SIGNALS

The discovery that selective chromatic adaptation may generate a variety of different colour sensations upon test stimulation at scotopic intensity levels seemed to imply that at least one of the basic assumptions of the duplicity theory was wrong.

Clearly, if one presumes that the scotopic contrast hues were triggered by cone impulses activated by the test light, one would be forced to accept that cone receptors may function at intensity levels down to the absolute threshold of the dark-adapted eye – this, of course, is in violation of the basic assumption that cones are less sensitive than rods.

On the other hand, if one presumes that the scotopic contrast hues were triggered by rod impulses, this would contradict the basic assumption that rods mediate achromatic colours only. On either presumption, therefore, the duplicity theory would have to be reformulated.

Evidence obtained in the 1960s and early 1970s favoured the second alternative that rods triggered the scotopic contrast hues, but its validity was first conclusively demonstrated by Stabell and Stabell (1975) when it was found that:

1. The spectral threshold and brightness curves of scotopic contrast hues coincided with the scotopic visibility curve (Fig 12.1).
2. Scotopic contrast hues could be obtained at an intensity level of nearly 3 log units below the absolute threshold level of dark-adapted cones.
3. Scotopic hues remained invariant of test wavelength and test intensity in accord with the Principle of Univariance.

On this evidence, the conclusion had to be drawn that the scotopic contrast hues were triggered by impulses originating in the rod receptors.

12.3 SCOTOPIC CONTRAST COLOURS DEPEND ON SELECTIVE CHROMATIC ADAPTATION OF CONES

The next important insight into the mechanisms underlying the scotopic contrast colours came when it was discovered that the disposition for the colour-related activity triggered by rod impulses was generated by selectively chromatic pre-stimulation of cones. Thus it was found that:

1. The scotopic contrast hue was approximately opponent to the hue of the pre-stimulation (Fig. 12.2).
2. The lowest intensity of the pre-stimulation light that could produce scotopic contrast hues was closely linked to the intensity level of the specific hue threshold of the pre-stimulation light.
3. Under simultaneous contrast conditions, scotopic contrast hues could be obtained when only cones were activated in the inducing field.

On this evidence the conclusion was drawn that the scotopic contrast hues were based on rod-cone interactions – that selectively chromatic stimulation of cones generated the disposition for the hue-related response triggered by rod signals (Stabell & Stabell, 1973a, 1978).

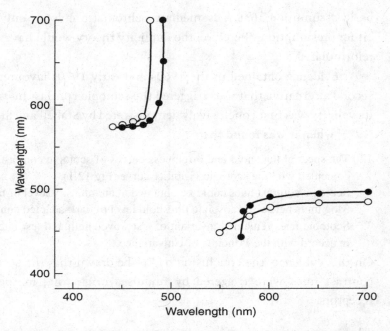

Fig. 12.2 Scotopic contrast hues (o) together with additive opponent hues (●). Abscissa represent wavelength of pre-stimulation while the ordinate represents wavelength of scotopic contrast hues. The field subtended 1 × 2° and was applied 6° temporally to the fovea.

12.4 SCOTOPIC HUES EXPLAINED

The conclusion opposed the basic assumptions of the Young-Helmholtz colour theory that the different receptor types functioned independently of each other, and that each receptor type mediated one colour quality only (see Helmholtz, 1896). The trichromatic colour theory, therefore, had little to offer as a theoretical basis of the scotopic contrast colours.

The question, then, arose of whether the conclusions could be explained more easily within the framework of Hering's (1878) opponent colour theory.

Hering had realized that colour vision must involve opponent colour processing somewhere in the visual pathway, but his phenomenological approach did not allow any conclusion as to the site of the antagonistic interactions. Three quarters of a century later, however,

Svaetichin (1953), using electrophysiological measurements, found evidence of a retinal origin. Thus, he obtained responses from cells in a fish retina that hyperpolarized for short and depolarized for long wavelengths. It was first assumed that these opponent colour responses were due exclusively to the cone system. Mitarai *et al.* (1961), however, provided strong evidence indicating that the rod system also contributed to the antagonistic colour responses.

The relation between the colour-related opponent responses of the retina and the pattern of discharge in the fibres of the optic nerve cells was later revealed by De Valois (1965). Recording from the lateral geniculate nucleus of the thalamus of the macaque monkey, they found cells which increased or decreased their rate of firing, depending on the wavelength. Maxima of excitation and inhibition were obtained in the red, green, yellow and blue regions of the spectrum in accordance with Hering's colour theory (De Valois *et al.*, 1966; Abramov, 1968). As with the finding of Mitarai *et al.* (1961), both De Valois (1965) and Wiesel and Hubel (1966) found to their surprise that the colour opponent cells also received inputs from rods under scotopic conditions.

With these remarkable findings and the evidence indicating that *hue* sensations were determined by the relative activity rate of the different types of spectrally opponent cell (De Valois *et al.*, 1966), the scotopic hue of successive contrast could be explained in a straight-forward manner based on the following assumptions:

1. Hue, both in scotopic and photopic vision, is encoded in the visual pathway by the relative activity rates of the different types of spectrally opponent cells.
2. The opponent cells are activated to about the same degree producing an achromatic sensation when the eye, in a completely dark-adapted state, is stimulated at scotopic intensity levels.
3. Following complete dark adaptation, selectively chromatic pre-stimulation of the three types of cone reduces the sensitivity of the opponent cells in proportion as they are activated.
4. Upon test stimulation at scotopic intensity levels, the change in sensitivity of the opponent cells produced by the pre-stimulation affects the impulse pattern initiated in the rods and thus changes the relative

activity rates of the opponent cells, giving rise to a hue approximately opponent to the hue of pre-stimulation.

The scotopic hue of simultaneous contrast was explained on the same principle. Thus, selectively chromatic stimulation of the three types of cone of the inducing field was thought to change the relative sensitivity of the opponent cells associated with the test area, producing a disposition for scotopic hue, triggered by test stimulation of rods (Stabell & Stabell, 1971c, 1973a).

12.5   MODIFICATIONS OF HERING'S OPPONENT COLOUR THEORY

As can be seen, this explanation of the scotopic contrast colours is in close agreement with Hering's opponent colour theory. However, when more specific tests of the theory were applied, predictions failed in several important respects, as clearly revealed in a series of investigations carried out in the early 1970s where wavelength, intensity and exposure time of pre-stimulation; wavelength and intensity of test stimulation; time between pre and test-stimulation; as well as retinal location of pre- and test-stimulation, were varied (see Stabell & Stabell, 1973a). Most importantly, pre-stimulation with primary yellow and primary blue colours produced, respectively, violet-blue and orange scotopic contrast hues instead of pure blue and pure yellow, as would be expected from Hering's theory, and pre-stimulation with primary red (obtained by mixing 700 nm and 470 nm lights) and primary green produced, respectively, scotopic green-blue and purple, instead of pure green and pure red. Presuming, in accord with the opponent colour theory of Hering (1878), that an intermediate hue sensation involved both pairs of the chromatic opponent processes and not just one pair, these results indicated that pre-stimulation with a primary hue generated adaptation effects in both the red-green and yellow-blue substances.

Also, the results showed that the scotopic contrast hue, although closely similar to the additive opponent hue of the pre-stimulation, was somewhat displaced towards shorter wavelengths in the 700–573 nm region and towards longer wavelengths in the 478–440 nm region.

Clearly, in order to account for the scotopic contrast hues obtained, the opponent colour theory of Hering would have to be modified, presuming that the points of equilibrium of the red-green substance (where no disposition for red and green is produced by pre-stimulation) were displaced towards wavelengths that had a red valence, while the points of equilibrium of the yellow-blue substance (where no disposition for yellow and blue is produced by pre-stimulation) were displaced towards wavelengths that had a blue valence (Stabell & Stabell, 1973a).

A similar criticism of Hering's colour theory had previously been presented by G.E. Müller (1930) who had suggested that 'Urfarben' may involve complex retinal processing (see section 5.2.8 and Fig. 4.1).

Hering's (1878) opponent colour theory also failed in another important respect. Thus, as noted above, Hering could not distinguish between achromatic scotopic and achromatic photopic colours. Hence, according to his opponent colour theory, one would expect scotopic and photopic contrast colours to be identical provided that (1) the pre-stimulation of cones was identical, and (2) the scotopic and photopic test-stimulations generated identical achromatic colours in a chromatically neutral state of adaptation.

This prediction was tested but not confirmed. Thus, the scotopic contrast colours, as compared with the photopic ones, were generally found to be somewhat displaced towards blue. This displacement was explained by the suggestion that short-wave opponent cells relative to long-wave opponent cells were generally somewhat more excited when rods, compared to cones, were test-stimulated (see Stabell & Stabell, 1994).

13   Rod-cone interactions in mesopic vision

13.1 ROD-CONE INTERACTIONS UNDER MESOPIC CONDITIONS IN A CHROMATICALLY NEUTRAL STATE OF ADAPTATION

In the period from Schultze (1866) to Lie (1963) it had been generally agreed that rods and cones interacted in a kind of colour-mixture process in mesopic vision. Rods and cones were assumed to contribute an achromatic and a chromatic component, respectively. The most advanced attempt to further characterize the rod-cone interaction under mesopic conditions had been made by Granit (1938, 1947) and Lie (1963). They both suggested that rod and cone activities antagonized each other at the retinal level in that the most sensitive receptor system tended to suppress the other. The rise of the specific-hue threshold obtained when rods intruded during long-term dark adaptation was compelling evidence in favour of this antagonistic interaction. There could be little doubt that rod signals completely suppressed the chromatic cone signals within the intensity interval between the cone-plateau level and the specific-hue threshold.

Yet, in apparent opposition to the psychophysical data and the hypothesis of rod-cone antagonism proposed by Lie (1963), the histological and electrophysiological evidence obtained in the late 1980s and early 1990s indicated that rods and cones *added* their responses of the same polarity both at the receptor and bipolar cell levels (Daw *et al.*, 1990; Schneeweis & Schnapf, 1995).

Fortunately, this apparent conflict between the psychophysical and the electrophysiological data could easily be resolved. Thus, the desaturation effect of the rods could be explained simply by suggesting that rod signals in a dark-adapted and chromatically neutral state of adaptation activated the different types of spectrally opponent cell to about the same degree. Hence, the differences in ongoing activity rates of the different types of spectrally opponent cells would become levelled down to some extent when light signals from rods intruded during the second phase of long-term dark adaptation (Stabell and Stabell, 1996). The rise of the specific-hue threshold obtained during the rod phase of the long-term dark-adaptation curve could thus be explained without invoking the retinal rod-cone antagonism hypothesis offered by Lie (1963).

This hypothesis of rod-cone antagonism was also challenged from another angle. Thus, quite unexpectedly, it was found that the specific-hue threshold for all spectral lights may fall well below the cone-plateau level when rod impulses intrude during long-term dark adaptation. Similarly, the specific-hue threshold of a monochromatic deep-red spectral light (700 nm) was found to fall markedly when an achromatic rod component was added to the 700 nm light in a completely dark-adapted state (Stabell & Stabell, 1971a, b, 1976).

Clearly, neither the hypothesis of rod-cone colour mixture nor the hypothesis of rod-cone antagonism proposed by Lie (1963) could account for the rod-cone facilitation found. Based on these hypotheses the specific-hue threshold level should never fall below the cone-plateau level when rod signals were added.

The unexpected rod-cone facilitation observed could, however, be explained by the following three assumptions (Stabell & Stabell, 1976):

1. Hue is encoded in the visual pathway by the relative activity rates of the different types of spectrally opponent cells (De Valois, 1965; De Valois et al., 1966).
2. Stimulation at intensities somewhat below the absolute cone threshold may excite a few of the cone receptors and, thereby, change the relative responsiveness of the spectrally opponent cells.
3. Rods feed spectrally opponent as well as non-opponent cells (De Valois, 1965; Wiesel & Hubel, 1966).

Thus, when, for example, the eye is stimulated with a monochromatic deep-red spectral light at intensities somewhat below absolute cone threshold, the light quanta might excite a few of the 'red' cone receptors and, thereby, increase the responsiveness of the red- and yellow-related opponent cells. If in this state rod activity were added, the relative activity of these opponent cells may be enhanced, and facilitate the specific-hue threshold. It should be noted that this facilitation of the chromatic cone component by rod activity could only be found under conditions where the chromatic cone component was relatively strong and the achromatic rod component relatively weak. Nevertheless, the conclusion had to be drawn that rod activity in a chromatically neutral state of adaptation was capable not only of desaturating chromatic cone activity, as previously assumed, but also of facilitating it.

13.2 ROD-CONE INTERACTIONS UNDER MESOPIC CONDITIONS IN A CHROMATIC STATE OF ADAPTATION

Ever since Schultze (1866) published his duplicity theory, scientists had inquired into how the rod and cone systems interacted in mesopic vision to produce a combined effect. As we have seen, the prevailing hypothesis had been that rods and cones interacted in a kind of colour-mixture process in which the cone and rod systems contributed a chromatic and an achromatic component, respectively.

The finding that rod signals also may give rise to chromatic colour sensations immediately raised the question of how rods and cones interacted when they both contributed a chromatic component.

A series of experiments was performed to explore this kind of rod-cone interaction. Three different procedures were employed: the change in colour of a test field was measured when (1) test condition changed from photopic to mesopic during long-term dark adaptation, (2) the rod stimulus was simply superimposed on the cone stimulus, and (3) light intensity of the test field was increased from scotopic to photopic intensity levels. Under all these conditions both receptor types contributed a chromatic component (see Stabell, 1967b; Stabell & Stabell, 1973b, 1974, 1998).

The results of the experiments indicated that rod activity under mesopic test conditions may contribute with all kinds of colour, and that the relative contributions of rods and cones in the colour-mixture process may change with test intensity, in that rods dominate at low and cones at high levels. Although this change in relative contribution was found regardless of colour quality of the rod and cone components, it could most simply be demonstrated when the rod and cone components represented a pair of opponent colours. For instance, when a blue rod and a yellow cone component were mixed and the intensity of the test field gradually increased within the mesopic intensity interval, the saturation of the blue rod component was seen to decrease gradually until only the achromatic component remained. Thereafter, the yellow cone component emerged with increasing saturation. Apparently, the rod and cone opponent colour processes antagonized each other to the extent that only the chromatic rod component could be observed at low and the chromatic cone component at high mesopic intensity levels. The inhibition of rods was completed when the test intensity reached photopic levels, where no trace of the rod component could be observed.

It should be noted that this inhibition of the rod influence has an obvious survival value. Thus, by taking over the control of the relative activity rate of the spectrally opponent cells at high mesopic intensities, cones may prevent rods from confusing the coded information about hue (Stabell & Stabell, 1973b).

Another fundamental difference between cone-cone and rod-cone mixture data was also revealed by experimental investigation. Thus, in sharp contrast to the cone-cone colour-mixture data, gross failures of the additive colour-mixture law were found when rod and cone colours were mixed. The extent of the deviation was found to vary both with colour quality of the rod and cone components, and also with test intensity (Stabell & Stabell, 1998).

14 Further exploration of chromatic rod vision

14.1 CONTRIBUTION OF J. J. MCCANN AND J. L. BENTON

Soon after the discovery that rod signals may initiate all kinds of hue, a number of research workers contributed to the further exploration of this phenomenon.

Firstly, McCann and Benton (1969) convincingly demonstrated that rods had the ability to interact with the long-wave cones (L-cones) and thereby produce a multicoloured image. This was illustrated by first illuminating a multicoloured paper with a 656 nm monochromatic light at an intensity level just above the colour threshold in order to activate only the L-cone mechanism. Thereafter, they superimposed a monochromatic light of 546 or 450 nm that activated only the rod receptor system. Adding the scotopic light dramatically changed the colour of the display; red, orange, yellow, blue-green, brown, grey and black could be seen in the display.

A more sophisticated and detailed study of this rod-cone interaction colour effect was later reported by McKee, McCann and Benton (1977). To produce the multicoloured display, a transparent photographic picture was taken both through a red and a green filter and then combined. The display was then illuminated with a red 656 nm monochromatic light at an intensity just above the colour threshold and by one of ten monochromatic lights selected from the 420–600 nm region of the spectrum. By increasing, in turn, the intensity level of each of the ten monochromatic lights they demonstrated that the threshold level of the multicoloured image (i.e. the lowest intensity level where the observer reported that he could see a faint image of red, yellow and blue-green) fitted the scotopic luminosity curve.

The intensity of the 656 nm light was then increased 1.2 log units and the observer asked to adjust the intensity of one of the ten monochromatic lights until the multicoloured image was judged to appear neither too red nor too blue-green. This judgement was termed 'optimum colour'. Under these conditions the observer saw a larger variety of colours, including whites, reds, oranges, yellows, blue-greens and browns. When the 'optimum colour'-threshold intensity was plotted as a function of wavelength, the curve again matched the scotopic luminosity function.

Lastly, a 510 nm light was directed either through the centre or periphery of the pupil while the observer adjusted the intensity of the 510 nm light to obtain 'optimum colour'.

The results showed that the 'optimum colour'-threshold was obtained at very similar intensity levels under these two conditions. Thus, the Stiles-Crawford effect associated with cone vision was absent, indicating that the 510 nm light stimulated rods only. On the other hand, a Stiles-Crawford effect became apparent when the intensity of the 656 nm light was further increased, so that the intensity of the 510 nm light reached above cone-threshold level before the 'optimum colour' threshold was reached.

The authors concluded that L-cones may interact with rods to produce a multicoloured image and that, therefore, rods may be as much a part of colour vision as cones.

A clue to an understanding of this remarkable ability of the rod receptor system was found in an observation made by McCann and Benton (1969). These authors had shown that when a *photopic* 495 nm test light was added to the 656 nm multicoloured display, the subject observed the same change in colour as obtained with the scotopic test light. The only difference was that the colours obtained with the photopic 495 nm test light appeared somewhat brighter, sharper and slightly more saturated. Accordingly, since the photopic 495 nm test light could reasonably be assumed to activate both the S-wave and M-wave cone receptors, McKee, McCann and Benton

(1977) concluded that rods may share the colour channels with both the middle- and short-wave cones.

14.2   CONTRIBUTION OF P. W. TREZONA

Another early contribution to the idea of chromatic rod vision was provided by Trezona (1960, 1970). Her starting point was an exploration of colour after-effects observed following stimulation with a 'white' stimulus (illuminant S_A). Retinal illumination, field size, time of exposure and the part of the retina stimulated were varied, and the subject, sitting in the dark, simply reported on the colour after-effects seen (Trezona, 1960).

The most significant after-effect observed was the so-called 'after-blueness' – a blue sensation that lasted only a few seconds. This 'after-blueness' was observable only when the 'white' pre-stimulation light had activated receptors outside the rod-free region. Hence, she concluded that it might be triggered by rods.

She found supporting evidence by reviewing previous studies where she, just like Willmer (1961), could point to observations that showed rod activity was associated with blue colour sensations under a variety of conditions. For instance, it had been found that when rod activity was added to a test field that matched the colour of a comparison field, a blue component had to be added to the comparison field in order to restore the match.

As mentioned above, König (1894) did not make any serious attempt to explain the change-over from achromatic to blue rod vision as intensity increased from scotopic to photopic levels. Trezona (1970), on the other hand, attempted to explain this shift in rod colour based on the assumption that rod signals had access to the spectrally opponent yellow-blue cells (the y-b unit), and that they would generate a blue colour sensation only when they reached above the threshold level of the (y-b) unit. Yet, she held that the 'blue' cones tended to inhibit rod activity and that, as a consequence, the blue-related rod activity would be increasingly inhibited as the intensity increased within the mesopic intensity interval when 'blue' test lights were employed.

14.3 CONTRIBUTION OF C. F. STROMEYER III

A third early contribution to an understanding of chromatic rod vision was provided by Charles F. Stromeyer III (1974a, b). He showed that the McCollough effect (i.e. a form-specific colour after-effect) could be obtained in scotopic vision. The McCollough effect was built up with square-wave gratings (0.75 cycle deg^{-1}), subtending an area of about 30 degrees square. In the first session the subjects were adapted for 20 min to a vertical grating projected in green light and a horizontal grating in magenta (red) light. The patterns were projected in alternate vertical and horizontal orientations and interchanged every second. A tiny fixation light was located in the screen's centre. After this adaptation procedure, the subject dark adapted for 30 min and was then test stimulated at scotopic intensity levels with a black-white test grating with retinal orientation and grating frequency that matched the adapting patterns.

The results showed that after adaptation to the vertical green and horizontal magenta (red) gratings, the vertical and horizontal test grating appeared faintly reddish and greenish, respectively, at the lowest scotopic test level, i.e. 1.8 log units below the cone-rod break measured for the white strips of the test pattern. Also, the subjects reported that the colours became more saturated as the test light was increased within the scotopic intensity range.

The experiment was repeated with a vertical grating projected in orange light and a horizontal grating in blue light. After this colour adaptation, the vertical and horizontal components of the white test pattern appeared, respectively, blue or blue-green and burnt orange or yellowish in scotopic vision.

To explain the McCollough colour after-effect in scotopic vision, Stromeyer (1974a, b) suggested that the adaptation to the coloured grating tended to depress sensitivity in cortical cells tuned to the adapting colour, spatial frequency and orientation. A test pattern similar to the adapting pattern would then produce less activity in these cells, and this reduced response would tend to signal complementary colours. Assuming that rod signals may feed into these cortical cells, the colour after-effect seen in scotopic illumination could be accounted for.

14.4 CONTRIBUTION OF S. BUCK AND CO-WORKERS

A more recent and systematic study of the effect of rod activity on colour perception has been performed by Steven Buck and colleagues. In a series of experiments, they attempted to single out multiple rod influences on hue (Buck *et al.*, 1998; Buck *et al.*, 2000; Buck, 2001; Knight & Buck, 2002). In the study, wavelength of a circular 8° test field centred 7° extrafoveally was varied between 420 and 630 nm in 10-nm steps. For each wavelength tested, the observers described the appearance of the test stimulus by using two of the four basic hues (red, green, blue and yellow) assigning a percentage to the relative strength of each component hue, so that the sum of the percentage equalled 100% for each trial. Following the determination of the hue percentages, the observers also assigned a percentage to the relative strength of the *saturation* of the test stimulus.

In order to measure the influence of rod signals on colour appearance, the colour scaling was obtained both in a completely dark-adapted eye and during the cone-plateau period of the long-term dark-adaptation curve, i.e. under conditions that, respectively, maximized and minimized rod contribution. The test intensity was mesopic, so that both rods and cones could be activated by the test stimulus when in the dark-adapted state.

Also, they measured time-dependent changes in rod influence on hue. A scotopic background field was flashed on for 2 or 6 s, while a mesopic test flash of 30 ms was presented at 1 or 5 s after the onset of the scotopic background flash (Knight & Buck, 2002).

Most importantly, the experiments performed provided strong evidence for a variety of different time patterns of rod influences on hue. Evidence was obtained for a so-called 'fast' rod influence that enhanced green relative to red and a so-called 'slow' rod influence that enhanced short-wavelength red relative to green and also blue relative to yellow.

Presupposing that rod signals had access to all three cone pathways of normal trichromatic colour processing, and that rod and cone signals acted with the same sign on shared neurons, they attempted to explain these different rod-hue biases on the assumption that the green rod-hue bias resulted from a stronger rod influence on M-cone pathways than on L-cone pathways, while the blue and short-wave red rod-hue biases resulted from a relatively strong rod input into S-cone pathways, i.e. pathways to small bistratified ganglion cells (Buck, 2004).

The basic assumption that rod and cone signals may mimic and reinforce each other was found to be consistent with a wide variety of psychophysical studies and also to be consistent with more recent anatomical and neurophysiological evidence indicating that rod signals, both through the primary and secondary pathway, are transferred to the cone pathway via gap junctions (see Fig. 10.1). Since gap junctions are sign-conserving synapses, signals from rods will tend to enhance cone signals both through the primary and secondary rod pathway (Daw et al., 1990).

Interestingly, the finding that the rod signals are transferred to cone pathways provides strong evidence that the cone receptor systems preceded the rod system in the evolutionary process and that the rod system simply utilized the already existing cone pathway in order to convey their information to the brain.

14.5.   CONTRIBUTION OF J. L. NERGER AND
CO-WORKERS

In a series of papers at the turn of the twentieth century, Nerger, Volbrecht and co-workers investigated the effect of rod activity on the unique hues of the spectrum; the pure blue, green and yellow (see Nerger et al., 1995, 1998; Volbrecht et al., 2000). The measurements were made both during the cone plateau period when presumably only cones were activated and in a dark-adapted state when both rods and cones were activated.

The results showed that the added rod activity in the dark-adapted state may change the spectrum locus of all three unique hues. Also, they found the rod effect to be most marked with small test fields.

To explain their results, they suggested that rods might contribute to both the R-G and Y-B opponent channels, and that there was a reciprocal antagonistic interaction between the rod and cone receptor signals. The reduced influence of the rods with size of the test field, for example, was explained by the assumption that the cones became progressively more effective in suppressing the rod signals as the size of the test field increased, in a similar way to their suppression when test intensity increased above cone threshold. They also attempted to explain the change in the spectrum loci of unique blue and green towards shorter wavelengths with rod intrusion on the assumption that rod signals tended to inhibit the short-wave cone input to the R-G and Y-B opponent channels (Nerger et al., 1995).

In summary, the study of chromatic rod vision made it clear that the two basic assumptions of the orthodox duplicity theory, that rods and cones function independently of each other and that rods mediate achromatic vision only, were wrong. Yet, it must be admitted that our understanding of the underlying mechanisms of chromatic rod vision is still in a rudimentary state.

Part IV Theories of sensitivity regulation of the rod and cone systems: a historical account

Introduction

The most basic assumption of the orthodox duplicity theory that only rods function in night vision and only cones in day vision has been generally agreed on during the whole developmental period from Schultze (1866) to the present (2009).

Schultze had provided two strong arguments in favour of this basic assumption. Firstly, rods and cones tended to dominate in nocturnal and diurnal species, respectively. In fact, some nocturnal species had a pure rod and some diurnal species a pure cone retina. Secondly, colour vision, a characteristic feature of cones of the central fovea, was absent in night vision.

Reasoning from this assumption, one would expect that a reduction in light intensity from that of daylight would lead to the functional appearance of rods at some particular intensity level. Schultze, however, did not state where and how this transition from cone to rod vision and vice versa happened. Furthermore, he did not provide any theory to explain the difference in sensitivity between the two receptor types. This reveals a serious limitation in his theory construction and shows that the most basic assumption of his theory was without any adequate explanation.

Several of the leading scientists within vision research have attempted to bridge this gap in Schultze's theory construction by developing theories of the sensitivity regulation mechanisms of the rod and cone receptor systems. Actually, the development of these theories may be considered a main thread in the history of the duplicity theory. The theories offered by Hecht, Wald, Rushton, Barlow and Lamb dominated the scene and will all be dealt with in some detail.

Early photochemical explanations

A first clue to an understanding of the sensitivity regulation mechanism in rods was given by the discovery by Boll in 1876 that the photopigment rhodopsin, situated in the outer segment of the rod receptors, was bleached by light and regenerated in the dark. He also showed that the bleaching effect of light depended on the wavelength used (Boll, 1878).

Influenced by this great discovery, Kühne, in an extensive research work, provided strong evidence in favour of the view that the sensitivity difference between rods and cones had a photochemical basis (Kühne, 1877a, b, 1877–1878, 1879). He investigated the bleaching and regeneration processes of rhodopsin in much more detail than Boll and made an important theoretical contribution with his influential 'Optochemische' hypothesis, where he presumed that the phototransduction in both rods and cones was photochemical in nature. Accordingly, he presumed that the apparent colourless cone receptors contained photochemical substances, and that these substances became involved in visual processing under daylight conditions. Indeed, in opposition to Schultze's (1866) duplicity theory, he presumed that even rods were activated by photochemical, colourless substances in daylight.

Furthermore, Kühne (1879) made an important distinction between the photochemical substances and their photoproducts, and argued that it was the photoproducts, not the photosensitive substances that generated the neural activity in the retina. Moreover, he discovered that rhodopsin may regenerate in two quite different ways: a rapid anagenese from photoproducts of rhodopsin and a slower neogenese from new substances formed after rhodopsin had been bleached. The relative contribution of these two processes was assumed to determine the speed of recovery of the rhodopsin pigment in the dark and, hence, the speed of the dark-adaptation process. Consequently, he suggested that dark adaptation would proceed most slowly when all rhodopsin molecules had been bleached.

The hypothesis that the photopigment rhodopsin could account for the sensitivity difference between rods and cones was apparently first unequivocally put forward by Parinaud (1885). He had found that 'hèmèralopie' reduced the sensitivity of the eye markedly and attributed this sensitivity reduction to the non-functioning of rhodopsin. In fact, he held that only the rod receptors had the ability to increase their sensitivity during dark adaptation and that the amount of rhodopsin determined the variation in sensitivity of the eye both during light and dark adaptation. He found confirming evidence in that the central fovea, which contained only cones, did not function in night vision, and that the photochromatic interval (the intensity interval between absolute light and chromatic thresholds) was nearly absent in the central fovea.

The final conclusive proof that the photopigment rhodopsin in the rods was responsible for night vision was given a few years later by König (1894) who showed that the spectral absorption of rhodopsin in humans closely coincided with the scotopic spectral visibility curve.

However, the suggestion of Parinaud that only the rods had the capacity to increase their sensitivity during dark adaptation was found to be wrong. Thus, Loeser (1904) convincingly demonstrated that the cones also had the ability to adapt to darkness. In fact, following strong bleaches he found that cones could improve their sensitivity by more than 1 log unit during the first few minutes of dark adaptation.

Contribution of S. Hecht

17.1 HECHT'S PHOTOCHEMICAL THEORY

The finding of Loeser (1904) that cones also had the ability to increase their sensitivity during early dark adaptation was confirmed by Hecht (1921/1922). He found that cones could increase their sensitivity markedly even during the first few *seconds* after bleaching.

More importantly, however, Hecht developed a photochemical theory for dark and light adaptation of rods and cones that had a strong influence on a whole generation of research workers. Certainly, he has played a central role in the developmental history of the duplicity theory. In a series of papers he provided an array of evidence supporting his photochemical theory (see Hecht, 1919/1920a, b, c, 1921/1922). In its essence and in its most simple version, the theory runs as follows: light acts on a photosensitive substance S and decomposes it into two precursors called P and A. The sensitivity of the eye, then, depends on the concentration of these precursors, not on the quantity of the photosensitive substance S. Thus, the model states that the amount of fresh precursors necessary for a threshold response is always a constant fraction of the amount of the precursors already present in the system. Hence, dark adaptation was thought to depend on the regular decrease in the concentration of the residual precursors present in the sensory system. This decrease was assumed to proceed according to the dynamics of a bimolecular reaction, to be independent of light stimulation, and, in accord with Kühne's (1879) 'Optochemische' hypothesis, to result in a reformation of the photosensitive substance S.

The fresh precursors, on the other hand, served to catalyze a simple chemical conversion of an inactive substance L into an active substance T, which then initiated the nerve impulse. The model was expressed in the following formulas:

$$S \leftrightarrow (P + A)$$
$$L|| (P + A) || \rightarrow T$$

in which $|| (P + A) ||$ means catalysis by P or A or both.

It should be noted that Hecht's (1921/1922) model for sensitivity regulation presumed that sensitivity variations during dark and light adaptation were determined in quite different ways. In both cases the sensitivity was assumed to depend on the amount of photoproducts P and A, but the mechanism that determined this amount was different for dark and light adaptation. During dark adaptation the sensitivity increase was due to the gradual and continuous decrease of the P and A material used in rebuilding the S substance, while, on the other hand, the concentration of P and A during light adaptation was assumed to depend on two opposing processes: a continuous increase due to the decomposition of the light-sensitive substance S when acted upon by light, and a continuous decrease due to the rebuilding of the S substance. Eventually, with constant light level, these two opposing processes were assumed to reach a balance or equilibrium, where sensitivity remained constant. If the light-adaptation level, then, increased, a larger amount of P and A would be formed by the increased action of the light, shifting the stationary state to a new point of equilibrium with reduced sensitivity.

17.2 SUPPORTING EVIDENCE OBTAINED FROM INVERTEBRATES

Hecht (1919/1920a) tested the photochemical assumption of the model by utilizing the light reflex of the siphon of an invertebrate animal (the common North-Atlantic long-neck clam *Mya arenaria*, a shelled bivalve mollusc). When the siphon of *Mya* is stimulated by light, it is shortened and its tip, thereby, moved toward the shell. The reaction time of this light reflex was assumed to consist of two distinct periods: a first sensitization and a second latent period. The first period was found to be of very short duration representing the time occupied by the necessary exposure to light. To test his assumption that this initial reaction of the light reflex was photochemical in nature, he investigated whether the sensitization process of the siphon reflex had the characteristics of a photochemical reaction. He measured the minimum light intensity necessary for a response to take place. *In each run* exposure time remained constant, but could be varied between runs.

Two quite different photochemical characteristics were investigated: (1) the well-known Bunsen-Roscoe reciprocity law where the quantity of light energy necessary to produce a given chemical effect is constant whether the intensity is low and the exposure long, or the reverse, and (2) the low temperature coefficient of photochemical reactions.

The results showed that the sensitization process of the siphon reflex of *Mya* followed the photochemical laws, and Hecht therefore concluded that it depended on a photochemical reaction.

17.3 SUPPORTING EVIDENCE OBTAINED FROM PSYCHOPHYSICAL EXPERIMENTS

Hecht, then, turned his attention to the adaptation processes of the human eye to explore whether his model also could be applied to human vision. At first, he found it necessary to supply the psychophysical dark-adaptation data already available with more accurate measurements. In particular, there was a need for reliable data on the rapid recovery of sensitivity during the first few seconds of *cone* dark adaptation. Just the extreme rapidity of recovery had made it difficult to obtain accurate measurements. In an important paper, however, Hecht (1921/1922) managed to make highly reliable measurements of the cone dark adaptation from the seventh second onward to the complete dark-adapted state. In fact, some less accurate measurements of the cone threshold were also obtained as early as two seconds of dark adaptation and by extrapolation backwards he estimated the threshold value at zero seconds dark adaptation.

The results obtained for the cones were found to closely fit a curve calculated from an equation of a bimolecular reaction. Since he had obtained similar photosensory behaviour both for the invertebrate *Mya* and for the *rod* dark adaptation of humans, he came to the conclusion that both cone and rod dark adaptation and the photosensory reactions in the invertebrate *Mya* could all be accounted for in terms of his photochemical model.

Yet, one important difference between rod and cone dark adaptation was stressed: while *threshold intensity* of cones measured during dark adaptation was assumed to be proportional to the amount of fresh photoproducts formed by the *test light*, the *log threshold intensity* of the rods was assumed to be proportional to this amount. Furthermore, presuming that this amount of fresh decomposition produced by the test light was proportional to the concentration of photoproducts *already present* in the sense organ, he could conclude that during dark adaptation:

$$T = kB \text{ for cones and}$$
$$\log T = c\,B \text{ for rods}$$

where T = threshold intensity, k and c = constants and B = concentration of residual P and A (see Hecht, 1919/1920c, 1921/1922).

Strong supporting evidence for the photochemical model was also obtained in a classical psychophysical study by Hecht, Haig and Chase (1936/1937). They measured the dark adaptation of the eye following light adaptation by utilizing a test procedure analogous to that employed on *Mya*. Thus, they used a test flash of short duration (0.2 s) and measured the lowest test intensity necessary to produce the threshold response. The major experimental variable was degree of light adaptation.

When the subjects were strongly light adapted (400 000 photons, i.e. troland, for 2 min), the cone and rod dark-adaptation curves were separated in time: the cone part started at once and was completed within a few minutes of dark adaptation, while the rod part showed up later and took more than 30 min to complete. They also found that the higher the initial light adaptation, the longer the eye required to reach a given threshold intensity during the dark-adaptation period, irrespective of whether cone or rod threshold was measured. Moreover, the dark-adaptation curves of the cones had a fixed shape. It was merely the vertical extent of the cone curves and their position on the time axis that changed, as if more and more of the same curve became apparent with increasing light adaptation.

Similarly, with strong bleaches, the rod dark-adaptation curves appeared the same, only moved along the time axis, as if the rod curve as a whole were moved to appear later the higher the light-adaptation level. Also, the curves of the three subjects closely coincided when shifted along the time and intensity axes, and only a slight day to day variation in threshold intensity for the same subject was obtained when the experimental conditions were strictly controlled. Certainly, all these results may easily be explained by the photochemical theory of Hecht presuming that: (1) the cone photopigments regenerate more rapidly than the rod photopigments, and (2) more photopigment is bleached as light adaptation increases. As a consequence, cone dark adaptation would proceed more rapidly than rod dark adaptation, and increasing light adaptation would produce more extended dark-adaptation curves, since more of the photopigment would have to be regenerated.

This simple photochemical view, however, broke down when dark-adaptation curves of rods at the highest and lowest light-adaptation levels were compared: The curves of the lowest adaptation levels proceeded much quicker than those of the highest levels. Apparently, rod dark adaptation could follow two different courses depending upon the level of pre-adaptation: a rapid and a delayed type. The delayed type was found to be established by light adaptation levels above 20 000 photons (troland) and the rapid type at levels below 200 photons. On this evidence they concluded, in accord with Kühne (1879), that the regeneration of rhodopsin may occur in two different ways: rapidly from the photoproducts and more slowly from new substances.

Contribution of G. Wald: photochemical sensitivity regulation mechanisms of rods and cones

This hypothesis of Kühne and Hecht must be considered an important insight with regard to biochemical processes underlying dark adaptation. Yet, it only represented a first step towards an understanding of the highly complex processes involved in the photochemical sensitivity regulation mechanisms of rods and cones. Obviously, a deeper understanding would require more information on both the molecular structure of the rod and cone photopigments and the bleaching and regeneration processes generated by light.

18.1 MOLECULAR BASIS OF BLEACHING AND REGENERATION OF PHOTOPIGMENTS IN RODS AND CONES

Inspired by Hecht, Wald, in the early 1930s, set out to throw light on these largely unexplored research topics (see Wald, 1949a, 1958, 1968). His profound discoveries and insights earned him the Nobel Prize which he shared with Granit and Hartline in 1967.

Firstly, he discovered vitamin A in the retina (Wald, 1933, 1934/1935). Shortly thereafter, he concluded that the photopigment rhodopsin was a conjugated carotenoid-protein engaged in a bleaching-regeneration cycle when acted upon by light (Wald, 1934, 1935/1936). Thus, in line with the hypothesis of Kühne and Hecht that light decomposes rhodopsin into its two precursors, Wald presumed that the carotenoids, all-trans retinal (vitamin A aldehyde) and vitamin A represented both photoproducts and precursors of rhodopsin.

A few years later, in 1937, Wald made two new important discoveries:

1. He showed that in addition to the red-coloured, well-known rhodopsin, there was yet another, purple-coloured rod photopigment which he aptly named porphyropsin (Wald, 1937a).

It turned out that the land vertebrates and marine-fish species possessed the rhodopsin system and freshwater vertebrates, the porphyropsin system, while species which could live both in fresh water and in one of the other habitats frequently possessed both photopigments, mixed or in temporal succession.

As might have been expected on this evidence, the chromophores (retinal) of the two rod photopigments were found to be very similar in structure. The principle difference was an extra carbon-carbon double bond in the porphyropsin chromophore (situated in the ring chain), displacing the absorption spectrum about 22 nm towards the red-end of the spectrum. It was also found that this change in structure was accompanied by very little change in chemical behaviour; the porphyropsin system constituted a bleaching and regeneration cycle of precisely the same form as that of rhodopsin (see Wald, 1937a, 1938/1939, 1949a, 1968).

2. Wald also discovered the existence of a *cone* photopigment in the chicken retina (Wald, 1937b). Obviously, the concentration of cone photopigments had to be very low relative to that of rhodopsin, since the outer segment of the cones, in general, appeared quite colourless. Wald, therefore, in his attempt to extract cone photopigments selected the chicken retina which contained mostly cones.

Firstly, he irradiated the retinal extract of the chicken with deep-red light (wavelengths above 650 nm) to which rhodopsin is relatively insensitive, and when the deep-red light produced no further bleaching effect, he exposed the residue to white light and thereby produced a renewed bleaching. The substances which bleached in the red and white light were assumed to be, respectively, cone and rod (rhodopsin) photopigments. The cone photopigment appeared violet in colour (maximum change in spectral absorption due to the red irradiation was obtained at about 570 nm) and Wald therefore named it iodopsin (visual violet).

In spite of the predominance of cones in the chicken retina, more rhodopsin than iodopsin was found. In fact, Wald estimated the concentration of iodopsin in single cones to be hundreds of times less than that of rhodopsin in single rods. Thereby, he could explain the relatively low sensitivity of cones and why cones had to be the organ of day vision. Also, he held that the Purkinje shift obtained with the chicken retina could be completely accounted for by a transfer from dependence upon the absorption spectrum of iodopsin in bright light to that of rhodopsin in dim light (see Wald, 1949a).

Wald soon concluded that the cone photopigment iodopsin, like rhodopsin and porphyropsin, was a conjugated carotenoid-protein. However, the important question of whether the same chromophores represented both the rod and cone systems or whether the chromophore of the cone photopigments represented a third variant of retinal remained unanswered.

At last, though, in the 1950s, Wald came up with a sweeping generalization (see Wald, 1958, 1968):

With regard to the molecular structure, all visual photopigments found in the outer segment of vertebrate rods and cones consisted of one of only two types of retinal (the rhodopsin variant retinal$_1$ and the porphyropsin variant retinal$_2$) bound as a chromophore to different proteins called opsins. Wald also recognized two families of opsin, those of the rods and those of the cones, so that, in all, four major photopigments could be synthesized in vertebrate rods and cones. Yet, in order to synthesize the visual pigments the retinal component had to be in a special shape, the 11-cis configuration. This configuration showed both a bend and a twist in the side chain of the retinal molecule which thereby fitted closely to the surface of the opsins.

Along with this parallelism of structure, the different visual photopigments were found to exhibit an extraordinary parallelism of the bleaching-regeneration cycle. We may summarize Wald's description of these two processes as follows:

The only action of light was to isomerize the chromophore of the photopigment from the 11-cis to the all-trans configuration (a configuration without the bend and twist, but containing the same chemical constituents). Since the all-trans configuration did not fit into the surface of the opsin like that of the 11-cis retinal, this transformation resulted in significant changes in the molecular structure of the photopigment leading eventually to a complete separation between the all-trans retinal and the opsin. A cascade of change took place. Pre-lumi-rhodopsin, lumi-rhodopsin, meta-rhodopsin I and meta-rhodopsin II all represented successive, stepwise, and rapid changes in the molecular structure before the compound was hydrolyzed, liberating all-trans retinal. Visual excitation had occurred by the time meta II had been formed (at about 1 ms), since subsequent changes were too slow to be involved.

Finally, the all-trans retinal was converted to vitamin A by an enzymatic process (retinal reductase as apoenzyme and DPN-H_2 as coenzyme) in which the retinal molecule received two hydrogen atoms from the coenzyme, reducing its carbonyl group to the primary alcohol group of vitamin A. Retinal$_1$ was reduced to vitamin A$_1$ and retinal$_2$ to vitamin A$_2$ (see Wald, 1949b). Later, it was found that other coenzymes may also be used in the enzymatic process (see Wald, 1968).

Up to meta II the all-trans chromophore remained attached to opsin at the same site. As long as this was the case, absorption of a new photon could isomerize the all-trans chromophore to 11-cis retinal and thereby immediately regenerate the photopigment. In fact, the absorption of a second photon by any of the all-trans intermediates of bleaching could re-isomerize the chromophore to 11-cis retinal and thereby regenerate the photopigment. Somewhat surprisingly, then, absorption of light may bleach as well as regenerate photopigments.

Yet, in accord with the hypothesis of Kühne, the photopigments were also found to regenerate after complete bleaching from the vitamin A stage. Thus, retinal was continuously formed in the dark by an enzymatic process in which vitamin A was oxidized by alcohol dehydrogenase (vitamin A$_1$ and A$_2$ were, respectively, oxidized to retinal$_1$ and retinal$_2$). Wald, like Kühne, knew that the pigment epithelium, a tissue lining the fundus of the eye and in intimate contact with the rods and cones, played a crucial role in the regeneration process, since the synthesis of rhodopsin from vitamin A did not occur in a retina detached from the pigment epithelium. The significance of this dependence was, however, unknown (see Wald, 1935/1936, p. 367). (Even today the transport pathway from the outer segment of the receptors to the pigment epithelium and back again, and the specific mechanisms by which the transformation from vitamin A to 11-cis retinal occurs are not fully known.) Nevertheless, Wald presumed that opsin trapped 11-cis retinal as fast as it appeared to form the visual pigment and hence regulated how much vitamin A was oxidized and visual pigments synthesized. In fact, Wald held that with different opsins went differences in both the kinetics of bleaching and regeneration, and in the absorption spectrum (see Wald, 1968).

18.2 SERIOUS CHALLENGES TO THE PHOTOCHEMICAL THEORY

Despite the great contributions of Hecht and Wald, the photochemical theory of adaptation presented did not gain general acceptance. The main obstacle was the well-known fact that sensitivity measured psychophysically by threshold intensity was dependent upon the size of the test field. This finding had generally been explained by assuming that impulses from widely separated retinal areas converged on common pathways and thereby increased the sensitivity. Thus, in addition to the concentration of photoproducts, this convergence factor based on neural summation might influence sensitivity during dark and light adaptation (see e.g. Lythgoe, 1940).

18.3 THE NEURAL FACTOR REFUTED

The view that neural summation influenced the sensitivity increase during dark adaptation was challenged by Hecht, Haig and Wald (1935/1936). The evidence they presented indicated that changes in sensitivity with test area were due principally, not to the change in the area itself, but to variation in the rod-cone composition of the test field. Hence, to explore the influence of area specifically as area of sensitivity during dark adaptation, it would be necessary to confine the measurements to retinal areas essentially homogeneous in sensitivity.

Wald (1937/1938), therefore, in a follow-up study, measured the dark adaptation curves with test fields of angular diameters of 1°, 2°, 3°, 4° and 5° at 15° and 25° above the fovea. The results, however, clearly showed that even in these relatively homogeneous regions, the sensitivity increased markedly with test area: at 15° a seven-fold lowering of threshold, at 25° a ten-fold lowering.

Yet, Wald (1937/1938) held that this increase in sensitivity with area did not contradict the photochemical theory, since it could reasonably be accounted for by the simple properties of a mosaic retina with a population of relatively independent units. His analysis of the measurements was based on the assumptions that (1) a threshold response involved the activity of a fixed number of retinal elements, and (2) throughout all portions of the homogeneous retinal field the percentage of such elements was the same. Thus, he presumed that in a series of fields of various sizes the threshold intensity obtained would always correspond to the activation of a constant number of elements, and that the number of elements would be directly proportional to the field area.

Based on these assumptions Wald (1937/1938) arrived at a relatively simple formula, which could accurately describe the change in threshold intensity with area:

$$(A - n_t)^k \times I = C$$

where A = area of test field, n_t = the constant number of elements for a threshold response, I = threshold test intensity, and k and C = constants.

An important feature of this model was the assumption that the mosaic character of the retina was transferred relatively intact as far as to the occipital cortex. Nevertheless, he did not preclude the possibility of some integration of the responses from the individual elements that could increase sensitivity somewhat. Such interaction, however, was assumed to take place somewhere in the brain.

The equation found for the extrafoveal test fields was also assumed to be valid for the central foveal area, where the constant number of elements for a threshold response (n_t) was presumed to be represented by cone receptors. Since in this case (n_t) was assumed to be very small, the threshold-area equation was reduced to the simple form:

$$A^k \times I = C$$

This presumption was supported by available data obtained within the central fovea.

The mosaic theory offered by Wald may be seen as a successful attempt to rescue the photochemical theory. Yet, there still remained a serious challenge to this theory. Thus, it had been found that the ordinary dark-adaptation curve proceeded faster and further as size of the test field increased, while the change in concentration of a photopigment during dark adaptation, on the other hand, would follow the same course irrespective of test size. Apparently, a neural factor had to be involved to explain the dark-adaptation process.

Wald (1958), however, argued that the change in sensitivity obtained was just what one would expect provided it was determined by the synthesizing of a photochemical pigment in a *large* number of receptors. Thus, one would expect the dark-adaptation curve to reflect, from moment to moment, the activation of a *sample* of the most sensitive receptors from a population of hundreds or thousands of receptors. Different receptors would then be involved in threshold determination at different times during the dark-adaptation period. Hence, the larger the population, i.e. the larger the test field, the further the dark-adaptation curve would be expected to depart from the adaptation curve of a single rod or cone, yielding a more rapid and extensive adaptation the larger the field.

19 Relationship between amount of rhodopsin and sensitivity during dark adaptation

On the discoveries of Boll (1877) and Kühne (1877, 1878, 1879) that rhodopsin in rods is engaged in reversible cycles of bleaching and regeneration, Parinaud (1885) had suggested that changes in visual sensitivity were due to variation in the amount of rhodopsin. This view had a great impact. Thus, for a long period it became generally accepted that the alteration of visual sensitivity in light and dark adaptation reflected changes in the concentration of the visual pigments and hence their capacity to absorb light.

19.1 RESULTS OF TANSLEY

Tansley (1931) appears to be the first to measure quantitatively the change in rhodopsin concentration during dark adaptation. She light adapted albino rats almost completely and then measured the quantity of rhodopsin extracted after varying times (from 2.5 to 1140 min) in the dark. The results obtained could be explained both by bimolecular and monomolecular reactions, although the monomolecular reaction was found to fit slightly better. In accordance with Parinaud's (1885) assumption, she obtained a striking similarity between the regeneration curve of rhodopsin of the albino rat and the dark-adaptation curve measured in humans. Hence, she suggested that the sensitivity during dark adaptation was proportional to the amount of rhodopsin present in the retina.

19.2 RESULTS OF GRANIT

This simple photochemical theory of dark adaptation, however, eventually met with serious difficulties. Thus, evidence put forward by Granit *et al.* (1938, 1939) strongly suggested that the amount of rhodopsin played only a minor role in sensitivity regulation during light and dark adaptation. In a pioneering study they made parallel measurements between the increase in sensitivity, as measured by the increase in the b-wave of the electroretinogram, and the rise in the concentration of rhodopsin during dark adaptation. Eyes of both frogs and cats were used.

Their results strongly opposed the hypotheses of Parinaud (1885) and Tansley (1931) that there existed a close and direct relationship between concentration of rhodopsin and sensitivity. Thus, they found a marked delay in the rise of the b-wave response relative to the increase in concentration of rhodopsin during dark adaptation. Indeed, the fast phase of the increase in the b-wave response did not start until the rhodopsin concentration had reached about 50% of the complete dark-adapted value. Furthermore, with frogs they found that when the b-wave was reduced to nearly half its dark-adapted value by light adaptation, the total quantity of rhodopsin had not changed by any measurable degree. Also, with decerebrated cats they found that when the b-wave was completely abolished by light adaptation, there was still 40% of rhodopsin left.

19.3 GRANIT'S EXPLANATION

To explain the lack of correspondence between change in size of the b-wave and the amount of rhodopsin during dark adaptation, Granit *et al.* (1938, 1939) suggested that inside the outer segment of the rods there was a bleachable store of photosensitive material which was incapable of initiating nerve impulses. Only a small fraction of the total amount of rhodopsin, situated on the surface of the receptor segment, was thought to be directly involved in the process of excitation. Illumination of this active material was assumed to initiate depolarization of the activated part of the surface and to give rise to the b-wave of the retina. The amount of photosensitive material available at the locus where the excitation took place was determined by the concentration of the 'inactive' rhodopsin through diffusion or otherwise. Hence, they concluded that the rate of 'diffusion' to the locus of excitation, not the time constant of the process of rhodopsin regeneration, was the significant factor for sensitivity regulation. The amount of rhodopsin in the store was only indirectly involved by participating in building up the excitable part.

Granit et al. (1939) concluded that their hypothesis could explain both the well-known delay of increase in rod sensitivity obtained psychophysically during long-term dark adaptation and the rapid and slow rod dark adaptation found when the degree of light adaptation varied (Kühne, 1879), i.e. all these results could be accounted for by. the rate of diffusion, but not by regeneration of rhodopsin.

The explanation of Granit, however, was rejected by both Lythgoe (1940) and Wald (1954). Lythgoe argued that each molecule of rhodopsin was a potential initiator of a nerve impulse when broken down by light, but that the final electrical response of the retina and optic nerve was determined by the existing synaptic arrangements. Accordingly, he regarded dark and light adaptation as two different processes where the receptors acquired, respectively, progressively more and less nerve fibres in common.

19.4 WALD'S EXPLANATION: COMPARTMENT THEORY

Wald (1954), in accord with Lythgoe, argued that *any* molecule of rhodopsin in a *completely dark-adapted* rod could excite it – each of the molecules was equally able to contribute to excitation. On the other hand, he accepted the finding of Granit that there was a non-linear relationship between concentration of rhodopsin and sensitivity.

To get a more accurate idea of this relationship, he measured both the percentage of bleached rhodopsin in cattle and the threshold level in humans during light adaptation. He found that when about 0.6% of rhodopsin was bleached, the corresponding threshold level increased more than 3 log units, i.e. more than a thousand times. This result was in accord with available evidence and clearly demonstrated that the simple photochemical hypothesis of Parinaud

(1885) was quite inadequate as an explanatory basis of dark and light adaptation of the visual system. Hence, a new theory was called for. To meet this need, Wald (1954) proposed his famous compartment theory of visual sensitivity regulation. The theory was intended to cover both light and dark adaptation for both rods and cones.

To explain the large rise of threshold when only small amounts of rhodopsin was bleached, he presumed that: (1) the rod receptor was a compartmented structure, (2) each compartment contained a considerable quantity of rhodopsin molecules, any one of which, on absorbing a quantum of light, would discharge the whole contribution of the compartment when the eye was in a dark-adapted state, and (3) the compartment could not contribute again until all of its rhodopsin molecules were restored.

Based on these presumptions Wald (1954) described the rise of threshold intensity by the formula:

$$n_0 / (n_0 - n_x)$$

where n_0 represented number of compartments in the rods and n_x the number of compartments that had absorbed at least one quantum of light. Hence, absorption of the first quantum of light by dark-adapted rods would raise the threshold $n_0 / (n_0 - 1)$ times. When half of the compartments had been discharged, the threshold would be doubled, i.e. $[n_0 / (n_0 - \frac{1}{2} n_0)]$, when 9/10 had been discharged, the threshold would have been raised ten times, i.e. $[n_0 / (n_0 - 9/10 \, n_0)]$, and so on.

Wald (1954) held that his compartment theory could explain both the discrepancy between the rise in threshold and concentration of rhodopsin and the delay of sensitivity increase during the dark-adaptation period obtained by increasing the proceeding light-adaptation level. Thus, the theory presumed that when one molecule in a compartment had absorbed a light quantum and discharged it, absorption of more light quanta would not raise the threshold further, but would tend to retard the subsequent dark adaptation, since the compartment could not influence sensitivity until its last rhodopsin molecule had been regenerated.

This last assumption could also easily explain the remarkable finding of Granit et al. (1938, 1939) that following high light adaptation, dark adaptation measured by the b-wave of the electroretinogram lagged markedly behind the regeneration of rhodopsin. Thus the compartment theory implied that light- and dark-adaptation threshold curves were related mainly to the bleaching of the first small fraction and the re-synthesis of the last small fraction of rhodopsin.

The compartment theory could also be applied to light and dark adaptation of *cones*. New considerations, however, had to be taken into account. This was because cones were assumed to possess very little visual pigment compared to rods. To illustrate the difference between rod and cone adaptation, Wald (1954) considered a hypothetical cone where each of the compartments contained only a single molecule of visual pigment. In such a cone each quantum absorbed would involve a new compartment and would result in a response. The sensitivity in such a cone receptor would, therefore, always be directly proportional to the concentration of its visual pigment, and the rate of dark adaptation would measure directly the rate of re-synthesis of the visual photopigment.

Hence, Wald assumed that the complication of light and dark adaptation of rods was due to the relatively high concentration of rhodopsin and that a simpler picture would emerge if concentration of photopigment were reduced, as in the cones. Indeed, in the limiting case, the simplest photochemical theory would apply: dark and light adaptation would follow in detail the concentration of the photochemical substance in the receptor.

Although Wald (1954) held that factors central to the photochemical systems of the receptors under special conditions could play an important role in determining visual threshold and adaptation, he suggested that under all ordinary conditions the photopigments in rods and cones were the major determinants – after all, he argued, the entire visual apparatus hung upon the initial action of light.

A few years later Wald (1958) attributed more weight to neural factors. Besides the obvious neural pupil factor, he also argued that the rapid phases of the adaptation processes could reasonably well be accounted for by neural factors. Hence, he admitted that both neural and photochemical components may be involved in light and dark adaptation. However, the relatively slow components of the adaptation processes measured psychophysically during long-term light and dark adaptation he still assumed were determined by the amount of visual photopigments.

19.5 A LOGARITHMIC RELATIONSHIP BETWEEN SENSITIVITY AND AMOUNT OF BLEACHED PHOTOPIGMENT

Substantial evidence in favour of this photochemical theory was obtained by comparing the rate of photochemical regeneration in solution and changes in visual sensitivity (see Wald, 1958). Thus, in accord with the rapid cone and slow rod dark adaptation obtained psychophysically in humans, he found the cone photopigment iodopsin in chicken to be formed at much greater speed than rhodopsin. Furthermore, just as frog and alligator rhodopsin was synthesized slowly and rapidly in solution, the course of rod dark adaptation of the frog and alligator, measured by the height of the b-wave of the ERG diagram, was correspondingly slow and rapid.

He found even more striking evidence in favour of the photochemical theory in results provided by Rushton and co-workers. They had obtained direct measurements of the fall and rise of visual photopigment concentrations in the human retina during light and dark adaptation by means of light reflected from the retina (Rushton & Campbell, 1954; Campbell & Rushton, 1955; Rushton et al., 1955; Rushton, 1957).

Wald (1958) pointed to three supporting results. (1) The steady state level of bleached rhodopsin in the living human eye by light adaptation was attained within about 5 min – about the same time it takes to completely light adapt the human rod system. (2) The re-synthesis of rhodopsin in the living human eye following strong bleaching displayed much the same course as the dark-adaptation curve of rods. (3) The regeneration of human cone photopigments, in contrast to the rod photopigments, was completed in 5–6 min, just as human cone dark adaptation.

Previously, Hecht (1919/1920c, 1921/1922) had given the photochemical theory an exact mathematical expression by assuming a direct proportionality between bleached cone photopigment concentration and sensitivity, and a proportionality between amount of bleached rod photopigment and the logarithm of sensitivity. Analyzing the available evidence, Wald (1958) concluded that visual sensitivity during light and dark adaptation in both rod and cone vision was logarithmically related to the rise and fall of the photopigment concentration.

19.6 CONTRIBUTION OF J.E. DOWLING

In his important 1954 paper, where he presented his compartment theory, Wald had calculated the relationship between amount of bleached rhodopsin and corresponding threshold level by comparing measurements of the amount of bleached cattle rhodopsin in solution and threshold levels in humans. Ideally, however, both types of measurement should be obtained from the same species.

Such measurements had first been provided by Granit et al. (1938,1939 see above) and were later applied by both Dowling and Rushton in order to formulate the relationship between threshold level and amount of bleached photopigments in mathematical terms (see Dowling, 1960; Dowling & Ripps, 1970; Rushton, 1961a, b, 1965a, b).

Dowling (1960) at first compared the b-wave threshold of the electroretinogram and the concentration of rhodopsin in rats on a vitamin A-deficient diet. Later, he made the same comparison in rats during long-term dark adaptation. Finally, he made a similar comparison between threshold measurements obtained during long-term dark adaptation and concentration of rhodopsin in the rod retina of the skate (Dowling & Ripps, 1970). Under all these conditions he found, in accord with the theoretical model of Hecht (1921/1922) that log threshold rose linearly with reduction in concentration of rhodopsin. The relationship obtained for the rat was expressed by the equation:

$$\text{Log } I_t/I_0 = 3.6 \ (R_0 - R_t) \ / \ R_0$$

where I_t and R_t are, respectively, the threshold and rhodopsin concentration in vitamin A-deficient or partly dark-adapted animals, and I_0 and R_0 are, respectively, the threshold and rhodopsin concentration in dark-adapted control animals. For the skate, he obtained a proportionality factor of 5.

19.7 CONTRIBUTION OF W.A.H. RUSHTON: RELATIONSHIP BETWEEN SENSITIVITY AND AMOUNT OF BLEACHED RHODOPSIN IN HUMANS

W. A. H. Rushton may be considered the leading authority within vision research in the 1960s and 1970s. His main interest was sensitivity regulation of the rod and cone systems. Shortly after Dowling's (1960) investigation, he addressed the extremely difficult task of determining the relationship between sensitivity and amount of bleached rhodopsin in humans (see Rushton, 1961a, b). Actually, he was the first to measure both the change in rod sensitivity during long-term dark adaptation and rhodopsin regeneration in the same subject.

In this endeavour he encountered a major obstacle in that cones are much more sensitive than the rods during the first phase of the long-term dark adaptation (Fig. 19.1). In fact, following substantial bleaching, about 90% of rhodopsin has regenerated before rod sensitivity surpasses cone sensitivity and hence can be measured below cone threshold. In order to overcome this limitation, Rushton used a so-called photanope as subject (i.e. a subject with deficient cone vision). Thereby, he could measure the change in rod threshold during dark adaptation over a range of nearly 7 log units (Rushton, 1961b). Using his densitometer, he also measured the regeneration of rhodopsin of the photanope. The relationship between the amount

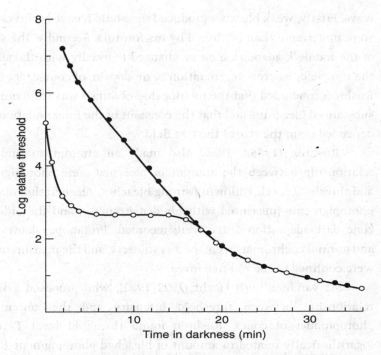

Fig. 19.1 Dark-adaptation curves of a rod monochromat K. N. (●) and a normal trichromat (o) following a full bleach. Wavelength of test stimulus was 550 nm; size, 1 x 2°; duration of exposure, 0.5 sec; and retinal location 7 ° in the nasal field of view.

of bleached rhodopsin and sensitivity during dark adaptation could then be calculated.

In agreement with Hecht (1921/1922) and Dowling (1960), the results from the photanope showed a close linear relationship between the fraction of rhodopsin still bleached and the logarithm of the rod threshold. The result obtained was assumed to be also representative for normal trichromats, since their rhodopsin regeneration curve and the last 2-log unit part of their rod dark-adaptation curve (the only part that could be measured in trichromats) coincided closely with those of the photanope.

Complications intruded however. Thus, Rushton found the simple linear relationship obtained to be restricted in two important ways. Firstly, weak bleaches produced threshold recovery curves that were more rapid than predicted by his formula. Secondly, the shape of the rod dark-adaptation curve changed markedly with the size of the test field, whereas regeneration of rhodopsin, of course, does not. Rushton concluded that the relationship obtained was valid only for substantial bleaching and that the constant of the linear relationship depended upon the size of the test field.

Rushton (1965a, 1966) also made an attempt to find the relationship between the amount of bleached *cone* photopigment and threshold level. Following strong bleaches, regeneration of cone photopigments (measured with his densitometer) and the ordinary cone dark-adaptation curve were recorded. Protanope, deutranope and normal trichromats were used as subjects, and the measurements were confined to the rod-free fovea.

At variance with Hecht (1921/1922), who proposed a linear relationship between threshold intensity and the amount of photoproduct of cones, Rushton found threshold level T to be logarithmically related to amount of bleached photopigment B. For the 'green'- and 'red'-related cone photopigments the relationship was given by the equation:

$$\text{Log } T = 3\,B$$

Unfortunately, due to the scarcity of 'blue' cone receptors within the central fovea, Rushton was unable to measure the relationship for the 'blue' cone photopigment (see Rushton, 1965a).

20 Post-receptor sensitivity regulation mechanisms

20.1 PSYCHOPHYSICAL EVIDENCE

The close relationship between amount of bleached photopigment and sensitivity obtained during long-term dark adaptation strongly indicated that the sensitivity regulation mechanisms were mainly located in the receptors. Both Hecht and Wald had accepted this basic assumption. Rushton (1965a, b), however, strongly opposed this view. Thus, he held that both the signals from bleached photopigments and the signals generated by background light regulated sensitivity centrally to the receptors in what he termed 'an automatic gain control-summation pool' (AGC pool). He based his position on two different lines of evidence.

Firstly, he found that a background light so weak that less than 10% of the rods could have caught a *single* quantum of light raised the threshold three-fold. Apparently, the 10% of the rod receptors that had received a single photon hit had markedly reduced the sensitivity of the 90% that were quite unaffected by the adapting light.

Secondly, Rushton (1965a) could provide strong supporting evidence in favour of his view by both light- and dark-adaptation experiments.

In the light-adaptation experiment, Rushton took advantage of an ingenious technique where he stabilized the light stimuli on the retina. The background was a black-red grating of period 0.5° (presumed to be less than the receptive field of the summation pool) and the test flash, a black-green similar size grating (presumed to activate rod receptors). The test flash superimposed on the background was alternately in- and out-phase.

The results showed that there was no threshold difference under these two conditions, supporting his view that the background light did not raise the quantum demand at the receptor level (i.e. the threshold for rod-receptor signals did not increase) and that all adaptation occurred at the pool.

This conclusion was also supported by experiments on dark adaptation where the bleaching light was sent by means of a brief electronic flash either through a grating of 0.5° period to give a striped bleach or through a neutral filter to pass an equal amount of light spread evenly on the retina. The test flash was under the latter condition a grating of 0.5° period, while it was an equalizing neutral test light in the former. Again, no significant differences between the two conditions were obtained.

Rushton (1965a) argued that if sensitivity regulation occurred at the receptor level, the dark bars of the grating should have shielded the retina from the flash of the bleaching light. The retina should thus have been fully dark adapted at the shielded regions, while every rod in the bleached area should have been substantially bleached when the same total bleaching light was evenly distributed on the retina. Hence, from his results he concluded that bleaching with the grating or with the same light spread evenly had about the same effect on the threshold level, and also that the threshold level obtained by the test flash was the same whether the test energy was concentrated by the grating or spread evenly – all in harmony with his AGC-pool hypothesis.

20.2 ANATOMICAL AND ELECTROPHYSIOLOGICAL EVIDENCE

Anatomical and electrophysiological evidence supporting Rushton's post-receptor adaptation theory was presented by Dowling (1967). Together with Boycott he had examined the synaptic organization of the retina in several types of vertebrate retina, including the primate, using an electron microscope. Striking support for Rushton's AGC-pool hypothesis was obtained. Thus, they found widespread reciprocal synapses between bipolar cell terminals and amacrine-cell processes. The anatomical evidence indicated that bipolar cells made synaptic contacts with both ganglion-cell dendrites and amacrine processes, and that the amacrine processes made synaptic contacts back on to the bipolar terminal. The amacrine cell was found to make such reciprocal contacts with bipolar cells over wide areas in primates. Also, the amacrine cells were found to extend their processes throughout the inner plexiform layer and to make synaptic contacts with each other.

The reciprocal synaptic organization found would obviously be suitable for a feedback system as required by Rushton's AGC model. Accordingly, Dowling (1967) suggested that activation of the amacrine process by the bipolar terminal might result in an inhibitory synaptic feedback on to the bipolar terminal, reducing the sensitivity of the bipolar cell in proportion to its excitation.

Dowling (1967) also found *electrophysiological* evidence in favour of a post-receptor adaptation site. Thus, he pointed to the study of Lipetz (1961, p. 639) who had found that illumination of one area in a receptive field of frog ganglion cells may raise the threshold in other areas of the receptive field – a result previously obtained in the classical study of the cat retina by Kuffler (1953). Furthermore, he found the b-wave of the electroretinogram, assumed to rise from bipolar cells, to be the first response in the visual system to show typical adaptation properties.

21.1 EACH RECEPTOR TYPE HAS A SEPARATE AND INDEPENDENT ADAPTATION POOL

Presupposing that the site of adaptation is located in summation pools situated centrally to the receptor level, one might expect that different kinds of receptor (rods, 'red', 'green' and 'blue' cones) would tend to interact in determining the adaptation process. In opposition to this view, however, Rushton (1965a) presented evidence suggesting that each class of receptor had a separate and independent AGC pool. Thus, he suggested that for rods and for each kind of cone the dependence of threshold on background and on bleaching were private, i.e. separate and independent.

Strong evidence in favour of independence between rod and cone adaptation pools was given by the well-known fact that the threshold level obtained during long-term dark adaptation may remain unchanged for several minutes during the cone-plateau period, while the sensitivity of the rods may increase by several log units. Indeed, with deep-red test light, the absolute threshold level of the cones may remain invariant for more than 20 min during the cone-plateau period before the rods eventually influence the threshold level. Furthermore, well-founded evidence in favour of the independence of the adaptation pools for *all* the different receptor types was found by Rushton (1965a) in the extensive research work of Stiles on incremental threshold (see Stiles, 1978). This research work may be illustrated by Stiles's well-known experiment together with Aguilar in 1954 on light adaptation of the rod mechanism. They briefly exposed a test stimulus in the extrafoveal retina superimposed on a steady, large adapting field. The threshold of the test stimulus was measured as intensity of the background field increased. They employed a blue-green test stimulus superimposed on a large red-adapting field to prevent cones from detecting the test stimulus. By this famous, so-called 'two-colour threshold technique', they were able to follow the incremental threshold of the *isolated* rod receptor system over most of its functional range before the cone receptors intruded.

Previously, Flamant and Stiles (1948) had provided strong evidence that the two-colour threshold technique could be used to isolate the rod receptor system. They had found that the reciprocal of the intensity of the adapting field required for different test wavelengths to raise the increment threshold by a fixed factor (1 log unit above the dark-adapted threshold) was very similar to the spectral sensitivity curve of the rod mechanism.

Stiles had obtained similar curves to the incremental rod curve under a variety of conditions intended to isolate the incremental curves of the different kinds of cone receptor. The results were judged to indicate that the different underlying adaptation mechanisms reacted independently of each other in that the most sensitive mechanism determined the threshold level except for a small probability summation factor operating when the two most sensitive underlying mechanisms approached equality (see Stiles, 1978). On this evidence Rushton (1965a) concluded that the different types of adaptation mechanism must operate independently of each other when threshold level is determined under light-adaptation conditions.

He then, in cooperation with Du Croz, investigated whether the different types of adaptation mechanisms also operated independently when threshold level was determined during dark adaptation (see Du Croz & Rushton, 1966). If so, they argued, it should be possible to obtain breaks in cone dark-adaptation curves similar to the breaks found in the incremental threshold curves obtained by the two-colour threshold technique and to the cone-rod break, by changing the relative sensitivity of the three cone-receptor types during dark adaptation. Their prediction was confirmed.

For example, bleaching the 'red' and 'green' cone photopigments completely with an orange light that was hardly absorbed at all by the 'blue' cone photopigment was found to favour the sensitivity of the 'blue' mechanism to such an extent that it could be measured in isolation with a blue test light during the first 90 s of the dark-adaptation period. Thereafter, the sensitivity of the 'green' cone mechanism was found to surpass that of the 'blue' producing a break in the dark-adaptation curve.

Similarly, by selective chromatic adaptation, breaks between the 'red' and 'green' cone dark-adaptation curves could be obtained, and isolated 'red' and 'green' branches could be plotted in their entirety.

On this evidence Du Croz and Rushton (1966), in harmony with Stiles's hypothesis that the four receptor-adaptation mechanisms acted independently in increment threshold measurements, suggested that they also acted independently of each other during dark adaptation. Thus, the apparent independence of the dark-adaptation curves found for the four receptor mechanisms was assumed to imply separate and independent AGC organization: for each of the four dark-adaptation mechanisms the threshold was thought to be determined only by its own photopigment and its own AGC pool (see Rushton, 1965a).

21.2 ARE LIGHT AND DARK ADAPTATION REALLY EQUIVALENT?

The similarity between light and dark adaptation found could easily be accounted for if they were based on the same underlying mechanism. To address this problem, Rushton made an extensive investigation to determine whether light and dark adaptation were, in fact, equivalent (see Rushton, 1965a).

The concept of equivalence of visual adaptation had been analyzed previously in a remarkable paper by Stiles and Crawford (1932) where they also put forward a test of equivalence: if two different adaptation procedures caused the same state of adaptation, then a given test stimulus should produce the same perception under the two procedures *irrespective* of the nature of the test.

The test of equivalence between dark and light adaptation had been carried out and confirming results had been obtained by both Crawford (1947) and Blakemore and Rushton (1965). Thus, both studies had found that variation in test parameters that produced marked changes in threshold level during dark adaptation produced the same changes in threshold level with light adaptation.

21.3 A DECISIVE EXPERIMENT

Yet, Rushton (1965a) was not quite convinced and therefore made an additional, so-called decisive test of equivalence, where he investigated whether the *spatial* organization of the adaptation pool for bleaching and light signals was the same. In this experiment, he measured dark-adaptation and incremental-threshold curves with the interposition of a perforated plate in front of both the bleaching and background lights. The holes of the plate were in sharp focus on the retina subtending an angle of about 0.5° from hole to hole.

The results showed that the dark and light adaptation produced vastly different adaptation effects: with dark adaptation, the log threshold elevating effect was found to be proportional to the average amount of bleached photopigment while with light adaptation the desensitizing effect (the increase of test intensity) was proportional to the average luminance of the background light confirming his general rule that the threshold is raised simply by the average light flux independent of spatial distribution (within the summation area) of the background light. Apparently, there had to be a marked difference between the spatial spread of the desensitizing influence of real and 'dark' light. Consequently, Rushton (1965a) concluded that light- and dark-adaptation processes were not equivalent.

To describe the two different processes, he developed his AGC model in more detail (see Rushton, 1965a, b). Thus, he assumed that the background-light signal when entering the input of the gain box became logarithmically transformed as indicated by Fechner's famous law:

$$S = k \log R,$$

i.e. magnitude of sensation (S) is logarithmically related to magnitude of stimulus (R). The transformed signal, then, was thought to be fed back to the gain box and to summate with the bleaching signal. Finally, this summed signal was thought to affect log threshold level linearly.

21.4 THE ADAPTATION MECHANISMS EXPLORED BY THE AFTER-FLASH TECHNIQUE

Rushton (1972) presented an important further development of his model of light and dark adaptation. Together with Alpern and Torii he explored the adaptation processes by a new ingenious psychophysical technique. Thus, they adapted the test field area by presenting a contrast light flash φ and a steady background field θ in a surrounding annulus area. (Another background field could be presented in the test area.) The light flash φ was presented shortly *after* a test flash λ had been exposed.

Both φ and θ were found to increase the threshold level of the test flash λ and, hence, to reduce the sensitivity of the test area. This reduced sensitivity was assumed to be determined by an inhibitory nerve signal N. Presupposing that N would remain constant under conditions where the test flash λ was kept fixed at a certain intensity level and reduced perceptually just to threshold level by φ and/or θ, they could vary intensity of φ and θ for a constant inhibitory N-signal, and by repeating this procedure for other fixed intensity levels of the test flash λ, they could establish the relationship between all the three variables. In this way they obtained the following formula:

$$N = [\varphi/(\varphi + \sigma)] \bullet [\theta_D/(\theta_D + \theta)]$$

where σ is the so-called semi-saturation constant, i.e. the intensity of φ that raises N to half its maximum, and θ_D is the intrinsic light of the eye ('dark light') that may be seen when the eye is in a completely dark-adapted state.

The formula was found to hold for a large range of N, φ and θ variations and was therefore considered to be of fundamental importance for the understanding of the adaptation processes.

One important achievement of the formula was that it provided a quantitative explanation of receptor saturation like the saturation Aguilar and Stiles (1954) had found for the rod receptor. Previous evidence had indicated that there existed a basic difference between rod and cone background adaptation in that the rod response saturated when only a small fraction of rhodopsin was bleached, while the incremental threshold of the cones could be followed to very high background intensity levels where nearly all the cone pigments were bleached and yet showed no upward turn away from the straight Weber law incremental threshold behaviour that would indicate the start of the saturation process.

Their formula, on the other hand, predicted saturation both for rods and cones. Thus the equation shows that however great φ becomes, N will never reach $[\theta_D / (\theta_D + \theta)]$.

They performed a test that confirmed the prediction: cone saturation occurred as expected when a background light was presented only briefly – at a time when the increment φ was flashed upon it. Thereby the bleaching of the cone pigment was slight and the threshold rise could be obtained almost uncontaminated by any impoverishment of quantum catching through bleaching. The reason for previous failures to obtain cone saturation was thereby revealed: cones at high background intensities bleach much more quickly than rods. As a consequence, in attempts to demonstrate cone saturation under background equilibrium or so-called steady state conditions, much of the cone pigment is bleached away so that the capacity for absorbing light quanta becomes smaller, limiting the adaptation effect of the background light.

An interesting extension of their data was obtained by *bleaching* the photopigment in the annular surround to various degrees. They could then compare the test threshold-elevation effect of bleaching and steady background adaptation procedures. No equivalence was found. With background adaptation the semi-saturation constant σ remained invariant, whereas with bleaching adaptation it increased. These results, then, further strengthen the suggestion that background and bleaching adaptation were fundamentally different.

21.5 LIMITATIONS OF RUSHTON'S PHOTOCHEMICAL THEORY

Previously, both Rushton and Dowling had provided strong evidence that long-term dark adaptation was controlled by photochemical processes. Both had found that log rod threshold was proportional to the amount of bleached rhodopsin, i.e. $\log T = cB$. Serious problems, however, soon became apparent. Rushton (1972) pointed out two important limitations: (1) rod responses to light could not be registered before 50% of the rhodopsin had regenerated (as Granit, 1938, 1939 had shown), (2) when the adapting light bleached less than 10% of rhodopsin, the threshold level was found to be raised and to fall far more than expected on the basis of the Dowling-Rushton equation during the early phase of dark adaptation.

Rushton (1972) and Rushton and Powell (1972a, b) attempted to account for these limitations in line with the conclusions previously reached by Donner and Reuter (1968). These authors had obtained results with frogs that suggested that accumulation of meta II (a photoproduct of rhodopsin not yet degraded to leave free opsin) caused rod saturation under light adaptation, and that the decay of this photoproduct determined the first rapid phase of recovery during rod dark adaptation. Similarly, Rushton presumed that meta II produced strong afterimages and caused the observed deviations between the Rushton-Dowling formula and the actual threshold measurements. However, about 5 min after a strong bleach, the amount of meta II and free opsin were assumed to reach a state of equilibrium and thereafter to be proportional to each other, so that they both remained proportional to the log threshold elevation. He found supporting evidence for the photochemical explanation of dark adaptation in that the threshold level during dark adaptation remained invariant as long as total bleaching exposure (the product of bleaching intensity and exposure time) remained constant, obeying the Bunsen-Roscoe law of photochemical reactions. Even under conditions where the bleaching intensity was above the rod saturation level, the results were found to be in accord with the Bunsen-Roscoe law.

Rushton's conclusion that the early dark-adaptation process was photochemical and not 'nervous' was also in accord with the finding of Donner and Reuter (1968) that the sensitivity regulation effect of meta II was restricted to receptors that contained this substance, that is, meta II did not reduce sensitivity of neighbouring rods that had not been bleached.

Background adaptation, on the other hand, was assumed to be governed by a neural mechanism. The plainest evidence supporting this view was still found in that a background so weak that only a small fraction of the rods caught a single quantum raised the threshold several-fold.

Rushton's (1972) conclusion that bleaching and background adaptation were governed by fundamentally different mechanisms (chemical and nervous) was in sharp contrast to the theories of Parinaud (1885), Hecht (1921/1922), Wald (1954) and Barlow (1964) who all presumed that light and dark adaptation were based on similar processes. His strong rejection of this view is shown by his forceful statement on p. 503,

> The nature of visual adaptation is an extremely complex question and our understanding of it received a mighty set back when Hecht and Wald used their outstanding force and eloquence to insist that everything depended simply upon the level of rhodopsin in the rods and the photopic pigments in the cones.

And further, on p. 512,

> Hecht was correct in his conjecture that the dark-adaptation curve was correlated with the regeneration of rhodopsin, but he was

never able to decide what the relation was. His insistence upon the hopeless attempt to make a single kinetic system explain such utterly divergent adaptations as that from bleaching and that from backgrounds has thrown the whole subject into a lasting confusion.

Not only the kind of mechanism of bleaching and background adaptation, but also their sites of adaptation were assumed to be different. Thus, Rushton (1972) had come to suspect that bleaching adaptation was mainly sensitivity regulation in the receptors, while background adaptation was mainly a signal scaling mechanism proximal to the receptors – possibly situated in the horizontal cells. He found supporting evidence in the immense number of receptor-bipolar junctions these cells connected to. On p. 505 Rushton (1972) made his position clear, 'For eight years I have hoped that the horizontal cells are Fechner scalors, and I still hope so.'

22　Contribution of H. B. Barlow

22.1　DARK AND LIGHT ADAPTATION BASED ON SIMILAR MECHANISMS

In contrast to the assumption of Rushton that light and dark adaptation were determined by quite different mechanisms, Barlow (1964) put forward the hypothesis that their underlying mechanisms were very similar; that the sensitivity regulation during dark adaptation was mainly determined by so-called 'photon-like' events. Thus, he presumed that the presence of bleached photopigment caused the receptors to show effects similar to those induced by light. Both the bleached photopigments and light increased the intrinsic noise level of the receptors. In fact, the effect of bleached pigments was assumed to add to that of light so that the separate effects of the two factors could not be distinguished at the receptor output.

22.2　BOTH NOISE AND NEURAL MECHANISMS INVOLVED

There was, however, a serious obstacle to Barlow's noise theory, since the expected square root law was not fulfilled in incremental threshold measurements. Thus, if a light flooding the retina elevated the threshold solely by virtue of the intrinsic noise level of receptors (i.e. the statistical fluctuation in the number of quanta absorbed) the incremental threshold should rise in proportion to the square root of the intensity of the flooding light (see De Vries, 1943; Rose, 1953; Barlow, 1957). Opposed to this prediction, however, it had been found that, over a large range of background intensities, the incremental threshold for a large test field rose in direct proportion to the background intensity (the Weber law). Only for small test targets and moderate background intensities were the expectations fulfilled.

On this evidence, Barlow had to conclude that, in addition to the noise factor, another factor was involved causing the threshold to rise faster than simple noise consideration would have led one to expect.

22.3 EVIDENCE IN SUPPORT OF THE NOISE THEORY

In 1972 Barlow re-evaluated his noise theory. He agreed with Rushton (1965a) that the relation between the amount of bleached rhodopsin and rod threshold during long-term dark adaptation was given by the well-known Dowling-Rushton formula ($\log T = c\, B$), and that the threshold level measured during the dark-adaptation period, therefore, was somehow determined by the amount of bleached photopigment. If this suggestion were correct, there had to be a very rapid increase of the desensitizing reaction with a rise in the amount of rhodopsin bleached; the reaction would have to depend exponentially upon the concentration of bleached rhodopsin. No mechanism that could explain this reaction had yet been demonstrated, but Barlow argued that the receptors were structures with a high degree of organization, and that, therefore, a small proportion of altered molecules might cause disproportionately large effects. Bleaching a single molecule might significantly change the condition of other molecules in its vicinity, and cooperative action of this kind might give rise to an exponential law (Barlow, 1964).

Opposed to the suggestion of Rushton, however, that the dark- and light-adaptation mechanisms were fundamentally different, Barlow stressed the similarity, suggesting that dark and light adaptation were equivalent processes. Thus, he suggested that receptors in the dark, containing a proportion of bleached photopigment, signalled messages indistinguishable from those caused by the illumination of the receptors. The so-called 'dark' and real lights, therefore, had the same adaptation effect; they both enhanced the noise level of the receptors and, thereby, reduced their sensitivity.

He found supporting evidence in the results obtained by Crawford (1947) and Blakemore and Rushton (1965), who had demonstrated that variation in the test parameters that produced marked changes in threshold level during dark adaptation produced the same changes in threshold level under light-adaptation conditions. These results, then, passed the test of equivalence put forward by Stiles and Crawford (1932).

Yet, Barlow found an even more striking confirmation of the noise theory in the results obtained by Barlow and Sparrock (1964). They had shown that when the brightness of a background light under stabilized conditions matched the brightness of the positive afterimage obtained at any particular moment during long-term dark adaptation, the incremental threshold level of this background brightness was the same as the threshold level measured during dark adaptation at that moment. This result, of course, nicely fitted the view that the positive afterimage represented 'dark light' equivalent to real light with regard to adaptation.

22.4 OPPOSING EVIDENCE

Barlow (1972) also considered evidence that opposed his adaptation theory. He found that although some of this evidence might be surmountable, important objections remained. Firstly, Rushton (1965a, b) in his so-called decisive experiment had demonstrated that bleaching the retina with an array of small light dots and adapting the retina with a similar array of luminous dots produced vastly different adaptation effects, indicating that there was a marked difference between the spatial spread of the desensitizing influence of real and 'dark' light.

This suggestion was further strengthened by Westheimer (1968) who found that real but not 'dark' light could produce the sensitizing effect first demonstrated by Crawford (1940). Thus, he found no evidence of sensitizing interaction between test spots and annuli composed of real and 'dark' light, respectively.

Also, opposing electrophysiological evidence had been forthcoming. Thus, Cone (1963/1964) had found that the latency of the b-wave of the rat electroretinogram was not affected equally by bleaching and background light, and Naka and Rushton (1968) had found that background light, but not bleaching, produced a steady hyperpolarization of the intracellular recorded S-potential.

Moreover, psychophysical measurements had shown that the log difference between incremental threshold curves obtained with large, long duration test flashes and those with small, brief test flashes was markedly reduced as background intensity was increased. Barlow (1972, p.10) concluded:

> Clearly changes of performance of this sort cannot result solely from photochemical bleaching or alterations of receptors, and must involve changes in the neural mechanism. The loss of summation ability at higher backgrounds is accompanied by improved resolution; it is as if the retina changed to resemble a finer grain film being operated at a faster frame repetition frequency at higher luminance.

Similar conclusions had previously been reached by Granit and Lythgoe (see Granit, 1947; Lythgoe,1940).

Thus, although his original theory had received striking confirmation from several sources, Barlow (1972) acknowledged that neural-adaptation mechanisms had also to be taken into account to explain adaptation processes.

Another potential complication was that the human retina contained both rods and cones and that the cones were of three different kinds. Yet, Barlow (1972) obtained a great simplification by accepting Du Croz and Rushton's (1966) suggestion that Stiles's 'red', 'green' and 'blue' cone mechanisms with regard to threshold determination operated nearly independently of each other, both under bleaching and background adaptation conditions.

22.5 SENSITIVITY DIFFERENCE BETWEEN RODS AND CONES EXPLAINED

In his summary paper, Barlow (1972) also attempted to explain the marked difference known to exist between rod and cone sensitivity.

Three different contributory factors were mentioned: (1) the 'dark light' of rods was generally much lower than that of cones, (2) rods had a much greater spatial and temporal summation capability due to the properties of neural connections between receptors and ganglion cells (by improving the conditions for spatial and temporal summation maximally, the relative sensitivity difference between rods and cones may increase by more than 1 log unit), and (3) the rhodopsin of rods had a greater total optical density than the cone photopigments. The latter factor, however, was assumed to play only a minor role.

23 · **Rushton and Barlow compared**

As can be seen, the theories of light and dark adaptation proposed by Rushton and Barlow disagreed both with regard to the site of the gain-determining mechanisms and the question of whether light and dark adaptation were equivalent.

In the 1965 version, Rushton held that the two processes were controlled in an AGC pool located centrally to the photoreceptors, while in the 1972 version he suggested that dark adaptation mainly occurred in the receptors and light adaptation in horizontal cells. In both versions he held that light and dark adaptation were quite different processes.

The noise theory of Barlow, on the other hand, presumed that light- and dark-adaptation processes were equivalent and located mainly in the receptors – that light adaptation mainly resulted from statistical fluctuation of photons of the background light, while dark adaptation was controlled by photon-like events, possibly originating from photoproducts as a stream of events fluctuating randomly like the photons.

24 The Dowling-Rushton equation refuted

24.1 CONTRIBUTION OF T.D. LAMB

The theories of Rushton and Barlow were very much alive in the 1960s and 1970s and dominated the discussion about visual adaptation. The most convincing defence of Barlow's view was published by Lamb (1981). He admitted that Rushton's theory had received stronger support from the scientific community, but argued that Barlow's theory could more easily be reconciled with known properties of the visual system. He supported his view by presenting three strong arguments against Rushton's theory: (1) intracellular electrical recording from rods and cones under conditions of light adaptation had shown that *photoreceptors* could become desensitized in a way approximating the Weber law, (2) Rushton's theory implied that the photoreceptor could generate two quite different signals: an incident light intensity signal and a signal of the fraction of bleached photopigment, but no distinguishing mechanism located in the receptor had been found, and (3) the uniform desensitizing effect found by Rushton and Westheimer (1962) and Rushton (1965a) could not be repeated in an experiment performed by Barlow and Andrews (1973). In fact, these authors found a marked difference between sensitivity in the dark and bleached areas.

Lamb (1981) then went on to propose his own specification of Barlow's theory. By analyzing a series of rod dark-adaptation curves of a trichromat previously published by Pugh (1975), he came to the conclusion that the long-term dark-adaptation curve of rods could best be described by three straight lines, each with a different slope. Furthermore, he suggested that these three different segments of the rod dark-adaptation curve were determined by the decay of three photochemical products S_1, S_2 and S_3. Indeed, he proposed a direct proportionality between threshold elevation and photoproduct concentration and, hence, suggested that the three different segments of the rod dark-adaptation curve were direct plots of the decay of the three photochemical products.

To account for the threshold elevation effect of the photoproducts, he presumed that they produced 'dark light' or 'noise' like a stream of photon events. Specifically, he held that the formation of a hypothetical photoproduct and activator S_0 determined the transduction process in the same way irrespective of whether S_0 was produced by photoisomerization, thermalisomerization, or by reverse biochemical reactions from the three intermediates S_1, S_2 and S_3.

In addition to the psychophysical evidence, Lamb (1981) could provide strong electrophysiological evidence in support of his theory. Thus, he had observed an increased fluctuation in the rod outer-segment current following a bleach. Indeed, the fluctuation had the form expected for randomly occurring photon-like events.

It should be noted that the photoproducts S_0, S_1, S_2 and S_3 are hypothetical constructs. The model as it stands, therefore, faces the problem of identifying and measuring the concentration of the four substances during rod dark adaptation and also of providing evidence that S_1, S_2 and S_3, in fact, are responsible for the three components of desensitization found in the rod dark-adaptation curves.

Yet, if correct, the theory of Lamb would provide an ingenious solution to Rushton's major problem of finding an explanation of the Dowling-Rushton equation. This equation had become generally accepted in the 1960s and 1970s, but since it required that the reduction in sensitivity was exponentially related to the fraction of pigment still bleached ($\log T = cB$, i.e. $T = 10^{cB}$), it could not be interpreted on a molecular level. Rushton *et al.* (1969, p. 473), therefore, had to admit, 'The threshold is raised very greatly by bleaching – in rods by about 1 log unit for each 5% of rhodopsin bleached – and we understand neither the mechanism nor the meaning.'

As we have seen, Lamb's (1981) solution to this problem was to suggest that the long-term rod dark-adaptation curve consisted of *three* different segments, each with a different slope, and that these three different slopes were direct plots of the decay of three different photoproducts.

Strong support of Lamb's assumption that the long-term rod dark-adaptation curve is best described by different consecutive segments was provided by Nordby *et al.* (1984) and Stabell *et al.* (1986b). Using a complete rod monochromat (K. N.) as subject, these authors could measure the sensitivity increase of the rod system during dark adaptation for about 7 log units and found, unexpectedly, that a major, middle part of the curve closely followed a straight line with a slope that was independent of size, exposure time and retinal location of the test stimulus.

Similar results were also obtained with trichromats (Stabell *et al.*, 1986a). The slope of the straight line component was found to be remarkably constant, not only in a given individual, but in different individuals as well. Hence, the evidence appeared to support the notion of Lamb (1981, 1990) that the normal long-term rod dark-adaptation curve consisted of several segments each with its own underlying mechanism.

24.2   THE SEARCH FOR A NEW FORMULA

The obvious next step was to relate the sensitivity change obtained during the middle, straight line part of the long-term rod dark-adaptation curve to concomitant change in amount of bleached rhodopsin (see Boll, 1877; Parinaud, 1885; Hecht, 1921/1922; Wald, 1954; Dowling, 1960; Barlow, 1964; Rushton, 1965a; Lamb, 1981; Pepperberg, 1984). By relating the psychophysical data of the rod monochromat and the trichromats to previous measurements of rhodopsin regeneration (Rushton & Powell, 1972b), a formula quite different from the Dowling-Rushton equation emerged. Thus, the results suggested that for both rod monochromats and normal trichromats the relationship between threshold elevation T and

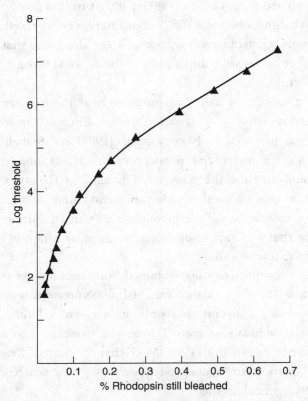

Fig. 24.1 Relationship between absolute threshold intensity of the rod monochromat K. N. obtained in the region of linear slope (wavelength of test stimulus was 550nm; size, 1 x 2 °; exposure time, 0.5 s; and retinal location 7° in the nasal field of view) and concomitant fraction of rhodopsin still bleached calculated from Rushton and Powell (1972). Time constant of rhodopsin regeneration adopted was 360 s.

concomitant amount of bleached rhodopsin B obtained during the major, middle part of the long-term dark-adaptation curve could be described by a power function:

$$T = c\,B^n$$

where c is a constant and the exponent n has a value between 3 and 4 (see Stabell & Stabell, 1996). (The exponent n of the power function could not be given an exact value due to the low reliability of the measurements of rhodopsin regeneration.) The relationship between the log threshold and the percentage of rhodopsin bleached with exponent 3.7 (time constant of rhodopsin regeneration 360 s) is shown in Fig. 24.1.

Actually, the relationship found between threshold elevation and the amount of bleached rhodopsin might also be valid for the rat and skate retina as evidenced by the results of Dowling and Ripps (1970). With these animals they obtained results corresponding to those of the rod monochromat in the region of 20–70% bleached rhodopsin by measuring concomitantly the b-wave of the electroretinogram and amount of rhodopsin bleached. Thus, the available evidence indicated that in this region a 10% regeneration of rhodopsin was coupled with a 0.5 log unit fall in threshold in humans, rat and skate, suggesting that the long-term dark-adaptation process was determined by variations in the amount of bleached rhodopsin, independently of interspecies variations in neural organization.

Since it was well-known that the electrophysiological (ERG) technique was relatively insensitive at low intensity levels, the marked difference between the electrophysiological and psychophysical data obtained during the last 20% of the rhodopsin regeneration period could reasonably be explained by the suggestion that the ERG technique used with the rat and skate did not adequately register the sensitivity change of the receptors during the last phase of the dark-adaptation process (Stabell et al., 1989).

24.3 DIFFERENCES BETWEEN ROD AND CONE DARK ADAPTATION

To investigate whether the new formula obtained could be applied to cone vision, a series of cone dark-adaptation curves was measured and compared to cone photopigment regeneration curves provided by Rushton and co-workers (see Stabell & Stabell, 1989; Stabell et al., 1990).

The psychophysical results revealed an interesting similarity between the rod and cone dark-adaptation curves. Thus, it was found that the long-term dark-adaptation curves of the cones, like those of rods, contained a middle, straight-line segment (Stabell & Stabell, 1989; Stabell *et al.*, 1990). Yet, the speed and duration of the middle sections of the rod and cone systems suggested that their sensitivity regulation mechanisms were controlled by somewhat different enzymatic processes. Thus, the relationship between threshold elevation T and fraction of bleached photopigment B for cones could be expressed by the equation $T = cB^{2.5}$ and for rods $T = cB^4$.

24.4 LIGHT AND DARK ADAPTATION ARE NOT EQUIVALENT

As we have seen, the important question of whether or not the underlying processes of light and dark adaptation were equivalent had not been settled (see Rushton, 1972; Barlow, 1972; Lamb, 1981, 1990). It was, therefore, of interest to attempt to test the equivalence hypothesis using the rod monochromat K. N. as subject (Stabell *et al.*, 1987). K. N. was considered an ideal subject for this purpose, since his light- and dark-adaptation curves could be followed for more than 6 log units. Relying on the regeneration curve of rhodopsin published by Rushton and Powell (1972b), both the relationship between the amount of bleached rhodopsin B and threshold level T measured during long-term dark adaptation, and the relationship between background field illumination I and incremental threshold level T measured during light adaptation were calculated.

The two functions were found to be vastly different: the relationship for the dark-adaptation curve was $T = cB^4$ and for the light-adaptation curve $T = I^{0.65}$. When tested for cooperativity by double reciprocal plots (so-called Lineweaver-Burk plots), the results showed that the dark-adaptation function was indicative of a positively cooperative enzymatic underlying mechanism, while the light-adaptation function was indicative of a negatively cooperative enzymatic underlying mechanism. These results, then, supported Rushton's (1965a, 1972) position suggesting that light and dark adaptation were based on different underlying mechanisms.

24.5 ALLOSTERIC REGULATION OF DARK ADAPTATION

The crucial question of how the power function obtained during rod dark adaptation could be explained by underlying molecular processes remained. At first, it was thought that the relationship had to be determined by an enzyme, but no ordinary enzymatic reaction that fitted the equation could be found. Soon, however, it was realized that the power function could be explained by the classical model of *allosteric* functions proposed by Monod *et al.* (1965) (see Perutz, 1989; Stabell *et al.*, 1986a, b, 1987, 1989, 1990, 1992, 1996).

According to this model (see also Monod, 1970), two states, an active R and an inactive T state, are reversibly accessible to allosteric proteins. Under conditions where a ligand has affinity exclusively for the R state, the fraction of the protein in this state is given by the equation:

$$R = (1 + \alpha)^n / L + (1 + \alpha)^n$$

where n is the number of identical subunits in the protein molecule, L (the allosteric constant) represents the ratio of molecules in the T to R states in the absence of ligand, i.e. $L = T_0 / R_0$, and α is simply a normalization for the ligand concentration (ligand concentration multiplied by ligand affinity for the R state).

When the allosteric constant (L) is very large (i.e. the intrinsic equilibrium is grossly in favour of the T_0 state), the equation can be simplified to:

$$R = c\alpha^n$$

where c is a constant.

Presupposing that this simplified version of the model of Monod *et al.* (1965) underlies the equation $T = cB^n$ found by Nordby *et al.* (1984), it was suggested that the concentration of bleached photopigment determined the displacement of the equilibrium between the active and inactive state of an allosteric, positively cooperative protein built as a tetramer (see Stabell *et al.*, 1986a, b, 1992, 1996).

This new model of dark adaptation presupposed that the cooperative effect of the bleached rhodopsin molecules giving rise to the power function was mediated by a conformational alteration (allosteric transition) induced in the enzyme molecule when it bound a ligand. The allosteric effect was thus assumed to be mediated entirely by the enzyme molecule and to depend upon its specific structure (Stabell *et al.*, 1989).

This intramolecular model of dark adaptation was opposed to previous photochemical dark-adaptation theories where the exponential effect of bleached rhodopsin was explained by assuming that bleaching a single molecule of rhodopsin changed the conditions of other rhodopsin molecules in its vicinity (e.g. Wald, 1954; Barlow, 1964).

24.6 A SEARCH FOR THE ALLOSTERIC ADAPTATION MECHANISMS

The close relationship between threshold elevation and amount of bleached photopigment obtained during long-term dark adaptation indicated that the middle straight-line segment of the long-term dark-adaptation curves was determined by photochemical processes. The question, therefore, arose as to whether there were allosteric, cooperative processes within the phototransduction cascade that might explain the relation found, i.e. whether a site could be found where signals from the bleached photopigment might affect sensitivity in an allosteric, positively cooperative manner.

By the late 1980s the phototransduction process had become fairly well understood (see for example, Fain *et al.*, 1989). Thus, it had been found that the absorption of light by the visual pigments in rods and cones triggers a cascade of biochemical events (Fig. 24.2). Firstly, the activated photopigment molecule diffuses within the disk membrane and activates molecules of the regulatory protein transducin. Each of these activated molecules, then, activates a great number of phosphodiesterase (PDE) molecules, which in turn, hydrolyzes a large number of cGMP (cyclic guanosine monophosphate) molecules.

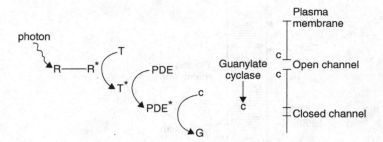

Fig. 24.2 Phototransduction. The enzymatic cascade that leads from the photon absorption of rhodopsin molecules in rods to the decrease in cGMP concentration is shown. Abbreviations: R, rhodopsin molecule; R*, activated form of rhodopsin molecule; T, transducin; T*, transducin in an activated state; PDE, phosphodiesterase; PDE*, activated phosphodiesterase; c, cyclic guanosine monophosphate; G, hydrolyzed c.

In the dark-adapted state, these molecules keep the membrane channels of the receptor open. Light, therefore, tends to close the channels. This light-induced closure reduces the inward cation current (mainly Na+) that flows through the channels and, consequently, tends to hyperpolarize the receptor membrane (see Fig. 24.3).

Since a significant amount of Ca^{2+} ions also flow into the receptor cell through the membrane channels when the eye is in a dark-adapted state, the closure reduces the influx of Ca^{2+}. This reduction in influx leads to a decrease in the intracellular Ca^{2+} concentration, since the extrusion of Ca^{2+} continues. Because Ca^{2+} tends to inhibit guanylate cyclase activity (the enzyme that synthesizes cGMP from GTP), the decrease tends to relieve the inhibitory effect of Ca^{2+} and, hence, to increase guanylate cyclase activity leading to an increase of cGMP (see Fain *et al.*, 1989) and, thereby, to a reopening of the membrane channels.

From this description of the phototransduction process the question arose as to whether *the membrane channels*, in fact, subserved the allosteric enzymatic function found for the dark-adaptation process. Biochemical evidence supported this suggestion, indicating that the opening and closing of the ion channels of the plasma membrane of the outer segment of the photoreceptor were,

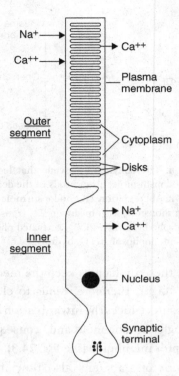

Fig. 24.3 Schematic diagram of the rod receptor illustrating circulating current. Only Na⁺ and Ca²⁺ are shown. Note that the stack of disks where the photopigment rhodopsin is embedded is separated from the plasma membrane.

indeed, controlled by an allosteric, positively cooperative protein. Firstly, Fesenko *et al.* (1985) discovered that cGMP, contrary to previous assumptions, bound directly to the cytoplasmic face of the ion channels of the plasma membrane of the outer segments of the photoreceptors and thereby regulated the transmembrane ion flux cooperatively. Secondly, from nucleotide sequence analysis of cloned DNA, Kaupp *et al.* (1988, 1989) attempted to identify the primary structure of the light-sensitive ion channel of the plasma membrane of the outer segment of the bovine retinal rod photoreceptors, and found that the functional light channel was an oligomeric protein complex, probably composed of four identical subunits, i.e. a tetramer, and that each subunit contained a single binding site for cGMP.

Strong evidence had also also been presented that only background light activated the cyclase activity (Matthews *et al.*, 1988; Pepe *et al.*, 1989; Kawamura, 1993). Hence, it was suggested that signals from bleached photopigment may control the level of cGMP in a reciprocal manner by their action on one or more of the biochemical steps linking photon absorption to the hyperpolarizing change of the plasma membrane potential without affecting the cyclase activity (Stabell *et al.*, 1992).

Light adaptation, on the other hand, appeared to be determined by the balance between PDE hydrolysis and cyclase synthesis of cGMP (Fain *et al.*, 1989; Fain & Matthew, 1990): an increase of illumination level would transiently lead to an imbalance in favour of the PDE hydrolysis. The reduced level of cGMP would then in turn be followed by an increase in cyclase activity, so that a new balance at a higher level would be obtained.

Yet, important questions remained. Thus, for example, it had long been known that calcium, in addition to its effect on guanylate cyclase activity, also had significant effects on one or more of the other biochemical steps of the excitatory cascade (Fain *et al.*, 1989; Nicol & Bownds, 1989). A detailed description of present day knowledge of the extremely complex processes and mechanisms of phototransduction has been given by Burns & Lamb (2004).

25 Several mechanisms involved in sensitivity regulation

A breakthrough in our understanding of the underlying mechanisms of dark and light adaptation of rods and cones would, of course, have represented an important step forward in the development of the duplicity theory. Yet, due to the complexity of the task involved, the progress in our understanding has proceeded at a very slow pace. Indeed, no general agreement about basic sensitivity regulation mechanisms of rods and cones has yet been reached (see Cameron *et al.*, 2006; Baehr *et al.*, 2007).

In line with Parinaud's (1885) assumption that both light and dark adaptation were determined by a changes in the amount of rhodopsin in the rods, most of the leading research workers during the hundred years that followed tended to conceive of adaptation as controlled by photochemical processes in the outer segment of the receptors. Of course, the research workers knew that this presumption was an oversimplification. Thus, it had long been known that sensitivity regulation of the visual system could not be controlled by one single mechanism operating at one site only, but rather was the result of different mechanisms engaged at different sites in the visual pathway. Besides the obvious regulation of the incident photons by the variation of the pupil size (in humans the diameter of the pupil may vary from about 8 mm in scotopic to about 2 mm in photopic vision, reducing the light incident on the receptors by about 1.2 log units), evidence had been provided indicating that important light- and dark-adaptation mechanisms were located more centrally than the outer segment of the receptors (e.g. Kuffler, 1953; Lipetz, 1961; Rushton, 1965a, 1972; Barlow, 1972).

Yet, the photochemical explanation of sensitivity regulation remained dominant for nearly a century. Gradually, however, evidence accumulated which clearly revealed that the photochemical theory was too elementary a conception. An early, important psychophysical study that challenged the theory was performed by Craik and Vernon (1941). They found that following light adaptation the ratio of thresholds of large to small test fields increased markedly with time in the dark, suggesting that the summation effect increased during dark adaptation and that the threshold curve, therefore, partly depended on an increase in the amount of interaction in the retina. Furthermore, by measuring the reduction of the brightness level of the positive afterimage with time in the dark following light adaptation, they could provide evidence that afterimages might also affect the threshold level and thereby influence the form of the dark-adaptation curve.

Strong psychophysical evidence opposing the simple photochemical theory of the adaptation phenomena was also provided by Wright in the early 1930s by his ingenious binocular matching technique. Using this technique he could measure the change in brightness and colour quality of a test light presented to the right eye fovea by a mixture of his three colorimetric stimuli (650, 530 and 460 nm light) presented to the completely dark-adapted left eye fovea. The changes of the test light measured were produced by pre-adapting the right eye to various coloured lights.

Summing up his results, Wright (1946) reported three different findings that clearly revealed that the photochemical adaptation theory was too simplistic.

Firstly, in cooperation with Walters, he found that his results did not obey the coefficient law. Thus, the effects of adaptation on two different test stimuli measured separately and then summed were significantly different from the adaptation effects on the mixture of the two lights. As an explanation of this breakdown of the coefficient law, Wright (1946) suggested that the three primary responses tended to interact in that stronger responses would tend to suppress or inhibit weaker ones.

Furthermore, by his so-called indirect adaptation technique, where the adaptation field was located at one side of the test field, Wright obtained extremely rapid regeneration rates, indicating that an electrical adaptation mechanism, acting 50–100 times faster than the chemical adaptation process, was also in operation.

Lastly, a quite unexpected observation was obtained when the 'blue' recovery curve of a blue (460 nm) test patch was recorded following yellow adaptation. Since yellow light would not be expected to activate the 'blue' receptors to any marked degree, one would predict that sensitivity to blue light under these conditions would remain relatively stable. Contrary to this expectation, however, he found an extreme reduction of the sensitivity of the blue test light immediately after the yellow adaptation (later termed transient tritanopia). Equally surprising, he found that, following adaptation to almost any radiation of the spectrum, a test colour chosen anywhere from the red-yellow-green range of the spectrum appeared to be admixed with a positive amount of blue. Even adaptation to a blue colour tended to produce blue when, for instance, a yellow test was employed. No blue afterimage that could explain the positive blue was seen in the dark. Hence, since the positive blue observed could hardly arise through any direct action which the test patch exerted on the 'blue' receptors, Wright (1946) suggested that the positive blue arose from a secondary reaction occurring upon test stimulation at a stage in the visual chain central to the phototransduction process.

Several research workers have later confirmed and extended Wright's findings . A particularly important and revealing experiment in this tradition was performed by Mollon and Poldon at Cambridge. They found that the sensitivity of a violet test flash on a steady blue background field *increased* 0.3–0.4 log units when yellow light was *added* to the blue field so as to yield a composite background field that appeared white (Mollon & Polden, 1979; Polden & Mollon, 1980). To explain this remarkable observation, they suggested that the blue background field reduced sensitivity both by reducing the gain of the short-wave receptors and by polarizing a putative, chromatically opponent B–Y channel. Hence, the added yellow light was assumed to reduce the polarization of the channel and, thereby, increase the sensitivity of the blue test light.

That the adaptation process may involve mechanisms central to the receptor level was also revealed by the so-called 'Crawford-Westheimer effect', the striking finding that when a small (typically 5 min) test field is superimposed on a background field that gradually increases in size, the sensitivity of the test field first decreases as the background field increases from 10 to 45 min, but then increases to a plateau level (see Crawford, 1940; Westheimer, 1965, 1970). Evidently, the site of the adaptation mechanism controlling the sensitization observed could not be in receptors (clearly, the sensitization mechanism did not operate on a spatial scale consistent with that of single receptors). The site might even be located central to the retina, since the Crawford-Westheimer effect did not show up in electrophysiological ganglion cell recordings (see Sharpe, 1990, pp. 92–95 for a discussion of its explanatory basis).

To add to this complexity, the well-known McCollough colour after-effect (a long-lasting colour after-effect specific to line orientation and spatial frequency of the adapting light, see Section 14.3) strongly indicated that the site of sensitivity regulation, under certain conditions, may be located at a cortical level.

26 Sensitivity regulation due to rod-cone interaction

Perhaps the most profound change in our conception of the sensitivity regulation mechanisms, however, came when it was realized that the rod and cone activities were not mutually independent, but that rod activity could influence cone sensitivity and vice versa. Anatomical, electrophysiological and psychophysical studies all contributed to this change in view.

Well-founded histological evidence in favour of the rod-cone interaction hypothesis was provided by Polyak's investigations of primates, summarized in Polyak (1941/1948). He discovered that, with the exception of the midget cone system, rods and cones were connected to the same pathways in the retina. Furthermore, he showed that the retina of primates was an extremely complex structure composed of a variety of different types of neural networks strongly indicating that the retina, and not just the brain, was involved in analyzing and synthesizing visual information.

More direct evidence in favour of rod-cone interaction was provided by Granit's ERG measurements. These results were interpreted to mean that rods and cones competed for 'a final common path' when excited simultaneously, and that the more active receptor types tended to exclude the other (see Granit, 1938, pp. 65–66).

Later on, Gouras and Link (1966) came to a similar conclusion. They investigated rod-cone interaction in Rhesus monkeys by analyzing the discharge pattern of ganglion cells connected to both rod and cone receptors. Their results showed that impulses from rods or cones arriving first at the ganglion cell would tend to block impulses from the other receptor type when these arrived shortly thereafter. When, for instance, rods and cones were activated simultaneously by a light stimulus, the faster cone signals would antagonize the rod signals and cut them off completely. Gouras and Link (1966) pointed out that the transitory inhibition they had found would tend to prevent rods and cones from acting in the same place simultaneously and, therefore, might play an important role in the apparent independence of the two receptor systems obtained when tested at threshold levels (see Stiles, 1978).

Yet, the investigation of Gouras and Link (1966) was followed by a long series of psychophysical investigations that established beyond doubt that the two receptor systems also interacted at absolute threshold level. A pioneer study was performed by Frumkes et al. (1972). After dark adapting the eye for 25 min, they presented an adapting flash and a test flash concentrically at 7° in the extrafoveal retina against a continuously exposed scotopic background. The wavelength of the adapting and test flash could both be fixed at either 420 nm (to stimulate rods) or 680 nm (to stimulate cones). In a different experimental series, the time interval between the adapting and test flash was varied.

In opposition to the generally held idea of rod-cone independence at threshold level, they found that there was a marked reciprocal antagonistic interaction between the two systems in that the threshold level of cones was markedly raised by rod activity and vice versa. Indeed, in accord with the relatively long latency of the rod system, they found that the rod adapting flash increased the cone-threshold test-flash intensity level later in time than the cone adapting flash increased the rod-threshold test-flash level.

A series of psychophysical studies on cone-rod and rod-cone interactions with regard to sensitivity followed shortly. Inhibition, facilitation, sustained and transient effects were found and explored (see Frumkes et al., 1973; Makous & Booth, 1974; Ingling et al., 1977; Latch & Lennie, 1977; Temme & Frumkes, 1977; Frumkes & Temme, 1977; Blick & MacLeod, 1978; Buck et al., 1979; Buck & Makous, 1981; Buck et al., 1984; Buck, 1985). Surely, the 1970s and early 1980s witnessed the final blow to the long-held idea of independence between the rod and cone sensitivity regulation mechanisms.

27 Modern conceptions of sensitivity regulation

During the last two decades the presumption that sensitivity regulation is basically controlled by photochemical processes located in the outer segment of the receptors has been replaced by much more complex theoretical conceptions. A recent review paper on gain controls in the retina by Dunn and Rieke (2006) gives an excellent illustration of this development. The authors argue that there are multiple retinal gain controls (i.e. adaptation mechanisms) that adjust sensitivity to different aspects of the light stimulus such as changes in mean intensity, variability about the mean (i.e. contrast variability) and spectral composition, and that the gain controls have diverse temporal and spatial properties, serve different functional roles and are located at different sites in the retina. Indeed, an additional dimension of complexity is introduced in that the gain controls are assumed to interact with other computations carried out in the retinal pathways.

In support of their suggestion that gain controls of the cone system may operate at different sites in the retina, they present evidence that both small and large steps in mean intensity and contrast may alter the gain adaptation level of ganglion cells, while only large steps change the gain of the receptors. Strong support in favour of the suggestion that gain controls may operate at different sites had previously been provided by Ahn and MacLeod (1993) and Yeh et al. (1996).

Dunn and Rieke (2006) argued that gain controls of the cone and rod systems must be fundamentally different, since the intrinsic noise of rods is several log units less than that of cones. This, of course, gives the rods the advantage of being able to operate at extremely low light levels, but the scarcity of photons absorbed by the rods makes rapid control of gain on the basis of signals from single rods impossible in night vision. Thus, the authors point out that less than 0.1 photon is absorbed per second per rod under so-called low to moderate scotopic light intensity levels and that, therefore, the rod system has to exploit spatially averaging of impulses from many rods in order to adapt rapidly to a change in light intensity at these levels.

The authors found behaviour measurements supporting the suggestion that at least one adaptation mechanism that may control the gain of rod-mediated signals operated in the rod bipolar pathways. In accordance with this suggestion, they could conclude from their own physiological recordings that the synapses between rod bipolar and AII amacrine cells were key gain-control sites at low light levels. These sites, they argued, would provide a unique opportunity for specialized processing operating exclusively on rod signals.

Yet, the review article of Dunn and Rieke (2006) leaves us with the impression that research on visual sensitivity regulation is still at a rather undeveloped stage. Obviously, much remains to be clarified. Thus, the different roles in sensitivity regulation played by the different types of receptor, horizontal, bipolar, amacrine and ganglion cells, and also by cells central to the retina, are still largely unknown. Indeed, in spite of the great effort to reveal the gain-control mechanisms of light and dark adaptation at the very first ion channels in the visual pathway (the cGMP gated channels in the plasma membrane of the outer segment of the receptors), there is at present no general agreement about these sensitivity-regulation mechanisms. A deeper understanding would require more knowledge about how dark and light adaptation change the amount of cGMP that gates the outer segment channels and how these changes are related to sensitivity measured psychophysically. The picture appears extremely complicated, since evidence indicates that retinoids (all-trans retinal, all-trans retinol and 11-cis retinal), phosphorylation enzymes and Ca^{2+}-binding proteins all may modulate the sensitivity (Dean et al., 2002; McCabe et al., 2004). Knowledge of such influences are, of course, essential for an understanding of the adaptation mechanisms of the rod and cone outer segment channels.

The long developmental history described here is obviously at odds with the common conception that the duplicity theory is a static, well-defined theory formulated by Schultze (1866). Instead, it shows that profound changes in the basic presumptions have been made and that the duplicity theory still is rapidly developing 140 years after Schultze's publication. Actually, we are short of a satisfactory understanding of how rods and cones are involved in *any* of the major visual functions. This clearly reveals the developmental potential of the theory: since all visual processes are triggered by phototransduction in rods and cones, there will be no end to the developmental history of the duplicity theory until we know, with regard to all major visual functions, the differences and similarities between the rod and cone processing, and also when and how the rod and cone systems interact.

Part V **Factors that triggered the paradigm shifts in the development of the duplicity theory**

In retrospect, it can be seen that all the classical theories in vision research with the exception of Hering's opponent colour theory were instigated by what may be termed observational facts. The theories of Newton (1671/1672) about light and colour, for instance, were triggered by his observation that the prismatic solar spectrum was rectangular in form.

Accepting the laws of refraction, he had expected the form to be circular. Yet, comparing the length of the spectrum with its breadth, he found to his surprise that it was about five times greater. He also found the two sides of the rectangle to be straight lines and the ends to be semicircular. It is important to note that Newton's observations did not result from an attempt to confirm or falsify the refraction laws. Instead, the observations were made quite accidentally.

To explain his observations, Newton initiated a series of experiments, testing various hypotheses and soon reached the famous conclusion that white sunlight was compounded of an innumerable number of different rays and that the colours of the prismatic spectrum were original and connate properties of these rays – all in sharp contrast to the generally held view that the colours of the spectrum were qualifications of the white homogeneous sunlight caused by prismatic refraction.

Schultze's duplicity theory was also based on observational facts. Thus, he arrived at his theory by combining two different sets of data. (1) Diurnal and nocturnal animals tended to have retinas dominated, respectively, by cone and rod receptors. In fact, some diurnal species had only cones and some nocturnal species only rods in their retina. (2) Night vision was achromatic.

Apparently, these facts were derived mainly from his own painstaking histological studies and Aubert's (1865) demonstration that saturation of colours deteriorated during long-term dark adaptation. Conclusive evidence that only rod receptors function in night vision was later provided by König (1894), who demonstrated that the spectral absorption of the photopigment of rods (rhodopsin) closely coincided with the spectral sensitivity of the human eye in night vision.

Perhaps the best illustration of how an observation may trigger a paradigm shift, though, was the unexpected discovery by Boll (1877) that the photopigment rhodopsin in the outer segment of the rods bleached in light and regenerated in darkness. Boll soon understood that rhodopsin had to play an important role in visual processing and therefore started an investigation of its photochemical reactions to reveal its secrets. This research was quickly followed up by Kühne who, during an intense research period (1877–1882), arrived at his general photochemical theory of vision, where phototransduction both in rods and cones was explained in photochemical terms. Accordingly, he postulated the existence of photopigments, not yet measurable, in the cones. In fact, he suggested that even rods in the light-adapted state, where rhodopsin was substantially bleached, contained undiscovered, visually active photopigments.

The trichromatic colour theory was also instigated by an observational fact. Thus, the trichromatic colour theories of Lomonosow, Palmer and Young were all based on the old and well-known fact that three different pigments mixed in various proportions were sufficient to produce all object colours. This fact, however, did not bear much weight, since, as Newton (1730) and later Helmholtz (1852) had made clear, the colour produced by pigment mixing depended on a subtractive mixture procedure making it impossible to control the kind of rays that struck the retina. Also, Helmholtz (1852) found that adding three *spectral* lights could not produce all spectral colours, and that at least five different primary retinal processes had to be postulated in order to account for human colour vision.

For a long period of time, then, the trichromatic colour theory was a speculative theory without any firm foundation. Eventually, however, a firm basis for the trichromatic theory was provided by Maxwell (1855, 1860). Taking advantage of Newton's principle of gravitation, he demonstrated, in opposition to Helmholtz, that three primary lights were, in fact, sufficient to match every spectral colour. Furthermore, in support of the trichromatic colour theory he demonstrated that protanopes had a reduced form of colour vision in that they lacked the 'red' receptor system.

In contrast to these four classical theories, Hering's (1878) opponent colour theory was not triggered by facts, but by ideas, i.e. by Spinoza's famous doctrine of psychophysical parallelism as applied to vision by Mach (1865). Thus, Hering immediately embraced Mach's psychophysical maxims and made them both the starting point and basic presumption on which his deductions about brain activities could be made.

Yet, it is important to note that the psychophysical maxims of Mach only represented the tool whereby the opponent colour theory could be built – they did not form any part of the theory per se. Thus, to develop his theory, Hering also needed an analysis of the colour phenomena. Here he could take advantage of Goethe's colour theory – especially Goethe's famous colour circle where primary colour qualities and opponent interactions could be found. The development of the opponent colour theory in detail and his strong conviction that his theory was correct were, however, first and foremost based on his own painstaking and keen phenomeno-logical analysis as regards colour mixing, successive and simulta-neous colour contrast, and also successive and simultaneous colour induction.

Given these important features of the development of the duplicity theory, the question naturally arises as to whether they

are representative of scientific progress in general. An answer to this
question presupposes knowledge about this progress – which has been
mainly explored within the philosophy of science. The contributions
of Popper and Kuhn have become classic (for an evaluation see
Chalmers, 1986).

28 Summary of K. R. Popper's and T. S. Kuhn's models of scientific development

Although scientific theories and laws of nature may never be proved in any definite way by *induction*, as Hume had made clear, Popper (1969, 1975, 1994) pointed out that they may be falsified on the basis of empirical evidence and purely *deductive* reasoning, i.e. the modus tollens deduction form of classical logic (see Popper, 1975, pp. 75–77). Hence, he assumed that scientific theories could be tested by attempts to refute them, and by selecting the most successful theories that withstood severe falsification tests, Popper believed that science could progress ever closer to, but never reach, the ultimate truth. The key to scientific development, therefore, according to Popper, was not the collection of observational statements, but the emergence of competing, falsifiable theories. Only by searching for falsification of theories and, on this basis, selecting the most successful ones, could science hope to learn and advance.

Popper's view of scientific progress may be summarized as follows: progress starts when a theory is refuted or falsified. This will create a problem for the relevant scientific community. In order to solve the problem other falsifiable theories are proposed. These new theories are then criticized and tested. As a result one or a few of the theories will prove more successful than the others, i.e. they may withstand severe falsification tests, may have greater empirical information or content, may be logically consistent, may have greater explanatory and predictive power, and may be more simple. Eventually, however, even the most successful theory will be falsified. When this happens, a new serious problem has emerged which calls for the invention of new falsifiable theories followed by renewed rational critique and testing – and so on, indefinitely, since the ultimate truth can only be approached but never reached.

Popper (1969, pp. 406–407) presented his view in the following simplified diagram:

$$P_1 \rightarrow TT \rightarrow EE \rightarrow P_2$$

where P_1 is a first problem, TT the tentative theories that are offered to solve P_1, EE the elimination process where the theories are exposed to falsification tests, and P_2 the new problem which emerges from the exposed errors of TT. New theories have then to be found to solve P_2 and so on indefinitely.

The account provided by Kuhn is quite different (see Kuhn, 1970, 1994). He sees scientific development not as characterized by a succession of falsifications, but by a succession of traditions, i.e. periods of normal scientific activities punctuated by revolutionary alterations.

His vision of the way science progresses may be summarized in bare outlines as follows: the pre-scientific period is characterized by disagreement and constant debate over fundamentals, like basic problems to be solved, methods, results and theories, making it impossible to get down to detailed scientific work. Eventually, however, this disorganization becomes structured and directed when a single paradigm, i.e. a theoretical framework or 'disciplinary matrix', is adhered to by a scientific community. The paradigm guides the scientists with regard to basic questions, methods and hypotheses that should be adopted. In this first 'normal' scientific period, scientists articulate and develop the paradigm through painstaking and detailed experimental research. The scope of the scientific knowledge is thereby extended and the precision of the scientific statements sharpened, but the scientists do not aim at unexpected facts and new theories, and when successful, find none. To bear the burden of this esoteric and time consuming endeavour, the 'normal scientist' must be devoted and uncritical of the paradigm within which he works. Indeed, a failure to solve a problem in his research tends to be seen as a personal failure, rather than as an inadequacy of the paradigm. Fundamental anomalies in the fit between nature and theory may be ignored, explained ad hoc to resolve the apparent conflict or set aside for future work, but do not lead to a renouncement of the paradigm.

Sooner or later, however, the paradigm becomes weakened and undermined by an increasing number of obvious anomalies. Some scientists may then begin to lose their confidence in the paradigm and may even openly express their discontent with it. More and more attention is devoted to the difficulties by more and more of the most eminent research workers in the relevant scientific community. Speculative and unarticulated theories that could point to fundamentally new discoveries may be developed. In fact, this period very much resembles the pre-scientific period. The time is now ripe for a revolution if an alternative paradigm not beset with obvious anomalies is available. Kuhn has likened the change-over from one paradigm to another to a conversion and a gestalt switch. Indeed, the choice of a new paradigm is seen as a decision to adopt a different native language and to develop it in a different world. The development, therefore, is not a progress toward an ultimate truth.

Scientists embrace a new paradigm for all sorts of reasons depending upon idiosyncrasies of autobiography and personality and not primarily on logical considerations. Thus, the kind of factors that prove effective in causing scientists to change paradigm is mainly a matter to be discovered by psychological and sociological investigations, although logical arguments are involved such as numbers and the seriousness of the anomalies.

The scientific revolution is over and 'normal science' can continue when the relevant scientific community as a whole has abandoned the previous paradigm and adopted the alternative new one – leaving only a few dissenters who eventually die out. Kuhn sees the old and new paradigm as 'incommensurable'. Thus, there are no plain logical arguments that demonstrate the superiority of the successful paradigm, since the fundamental premises of the two paradigms are different. The decision to change paradigms depends in the last instance on the importance given to a variety of values, often in conflict, by individual scientists. The possibility of solving new puzzles that may please their institutions and promote their career may have a strong impact. No specific plan guiding the scientific development is apparent and no ultimate truth is approached.

29 The development of the duplicity theory as a test of Popper's and Kuhn's models

It is apparent that neither of these models fit well with our description of the development of the duplicity theory. As regards Popper's model, none of the classical theories of Newton, Young, Schultze, Kühne and Hering was triggered by an attempt to falsify or refute current hypotheses or theories. Newton's starting point was the rectangular form of the prismatic solar spectrum he observed when he looked at its beautiful colours; Young based his theory on the old and well-known fact that three pigments were sufficient to produce every object colour; Schultze reflected on the fact that nocturnal and diurnal animals tended to have rod- and cone-dominated retinas, respectively, and that colours were absent in night vision; Kühne's theory was instigated by the great discovery of Boll that rhodopsin bleached in light and regenerated in the dark; and Hering was spurred on by Mach's psychophysical maxim. Thus, there is little evidence of long, fruitful falsification periods ending with falsification of the most successful hypothesis and the development of a new, better one triggered by this last falsification.

It is evident that Maxwell (1855, 1860) provided conclusive evidence in support of Young's trichromatic colour theory by demonstrating that three standard spectral lights were sufficient to produce all spectral colours, but his experiments represented a *confirmation* of an already existing theory and not a falsification. It should also be noted that Young's theory was immediately accepted by the relevant scientific community without much debate following the discoveries of Maxwell.

Interestingly, the spectro-photometric measurements of Marks *et al.* (1964) and Brown & Wald (1964) that demonstrated the existence of three different cone photopigments situated in different cones have resulted in a transformation of the basic assumption of Young's colour theory from a theoretical to a *factual* status. There is, of course, no room for such a transformation in Popper's model.

Our description of the development of the duplicity theory is not easily reconciled with Kuhn's model either. Thus, in apparent contrast to Kuhn's account of scientific progress, the development of the duplicity theory has been marked by a series of important steps that all still are regarded as milestones in our understanding of visual phenomena. In fact, no so-called crises and revolutions, where one paradigm is abandoned and another adopted, are apparent. Instead, the steps taken appear to complement each other and may therefore exist simultaneously. Of course, an understanding of Kuhn's model depends to a large extent on how the concept 'paradigm' is interpreted. Yet, even if it is asserted that there has been no paradigm shift in vision research since Newton, one would have to admit that great discoveries and large progressive steps in the development of the duplicity theory have occurred and that, therefore, his characteristics of so-called 'normal science' would not be met. Also, the sharp differences in opinion between Hecht, Wald, Rushton, Barlow and Lamb in the twentieth century, where relatively little fundamental change has occurred in the development of the duplicity theory (and on these grounds might be characterized as a 'normal' scientific period), are not in accord with Kuhn's description where he emphasizes an uncritical and devoted attitude toward the ruling paradigm. Instead, the leading authorities have attempted to build their own theories on rational grounds, mainly in conflict with each other. Similar considerations apply for the period between Newton and Young.

Moreover, there is at present no indication that a single paradigm will emerge and dominate vision research. Contrary to this view, the scientific progress in vision research appears to move simultaneously in several different directions, focusing on visual processing at various stages between the retina and the central brain areas, on normal and abnormal processing, genetic problems and visual processing in different species. Thus, the number of subjects appears to increase with a continuing proliferation of scientific specialties, giving the impression that the scientific progress is diverging, not converging. Certainly, there is, at present, no sign that vision research will settle on a common paradigm.

Yet, the best illustration of the failure of Kuhn's model to provide an adequate account of the development of science, in general, is the paradigm shift from the presumptions of the Ancient Greeks (that the crystalline lens was the actual sense organ and that the information about the outer world was obtained by rays that emanated *from* the eye *towards* the object) to the conceptions of Kepler and Newton that the lens was just an optical focusing device and that light moved in the opposite direction. Obviously, this change in view is not merely a 'conversion' or a 'different language developed in a different world', but a change from false presumptions to assumptions that today are generally considered as facts.

As seen, Kuhn's model, like Popper's, gives no room for such a progressive change, also witnessed by the change in the status of Young's trichromatic theory.

It is apparent that the models of Popper and Kuhn have left out some important factors involved in the development of scientific theories. Perhaps the most important weakness of the models is that they do not give any adequate account of how *new* theories arrive. In the development of the duplicity theory explorations and unexpected observations not based on attempts to falsify existing theories (Popper) or triggered by obvious anomalies (Kuhn) have played a crucial role.

The question has often been raised as to whether scientific progress is mainly a rational process as assumed by Popper or an irrational process as assumed by Kuhn. The development of the duplicity theory obviously favours the assumption of a rational process. Such a rational attitude is well illustrated in Helmholtz

(1867) where he abandoned his own hypothesis and immediately accepted Maxwell's results and conclusions and, hence, the trichromatic colour theory.

Also, the dispute between the followers of Hering and Helmholtz was soon settled in a fruitful and rational way by the assumption that the Young-Maxwell-Helmholtz colour theory applied to early phototransduction processing in the retina, while Hering's theory applied to more central processing.

In fact, the hypothesis that the normal human retina contains three different kinds of cone, each with a different photopigment that absorbs light and, thereby, gives rise to a cascade of photochemical processes in the receptors that triggers neural processes, which at later stages in the visual pathway are transformed into opponent processing, is today generally accepted as a fact.

Thus, although Popper and Kuhn may be right in that science never will disclose the ultimate truth, scientific development entails the promising possibility that a theory may become attached to an increasing number of facts with increasing precision and ultimately be regarded as a fact in itself with important theoretical and practical implications.

References

Abramov, I. (1968). Further analysis of the responses of LGN cells. *Journal of the Optical Society of America*, **58**, 574–579.

Aguilar, M. & Stiles, W.S. (1954). Saturation of the rod mechanism of the retina at high levels of stimulation. *Optica Acta*, **1**, 59–65.

Ahn, S.J. & MacLeod, I.A. (1993). Link-specific adaptation in the luminance and chromatic channels. *Vision Research*, **33**, 2271–2286.

Aubert, H. (1865). *Physiologie der Netzhaut*. Morgenstern: Breslau.

Baehr, W., Karan, S., Maeda, T. *et al.* (2007). The function of guanylate cyclase 1 and guanylate cyclase 2 in rod and cone photoreceptors. *Journal of Biological Chemistry*, **282**, 8837–8847.

Barlow, H.B. (1957). Increment thresholds at low intensities considered as signal/noise discriminations. *Journal of Physiology*, **136**, 469–488.

Barlow, H.B. (1964). Dark-adaptation: a new hypothesis. *Vision Research*, **4**, 47–58.

Barlow, H.B. (1972). Dark and light adaptation: psychophysics. In *Handbook of Sensory Physiology, vol. VII/4 Visual Psychophysics*. D. Jameson & L.M. Hurvich, eds. Berlin: Springer, pp. 1–28.

Barlow, H.B. & Andrews, D.P. (1973). The site at which rhodopsin bleaching raises scotopic threshold. *Vision Research*, **13**, 903–908.

Barlow, H.B., Fitzhugh, R. & Kuffler, S.W. (1957). Change of organization in the receptive fields of the cat's retina during dark adaptation. *Journal of Physiology*, **137**, 338–354.

Barlow, H.B. & Sparrock, J.M. (1964). The role of afterimages in dark adaptation. *Science*, **144**, 1309–1314.

Blakemore, C.B. & Rushton, W.A.H. (1965). Dark adaptation and increment threshold in a rod monochromat. *Journal of Physiology*, London, **181**, 612–628.

Blanchard, J. (1918). The brightness sensibility of the retina. *Physical Review*, **11**, 81–99.

Blick, D.W. & MacLeod, D.I.A. (1978). Rod threshold: influence of neighboring cones. *Vision Research*, **18**, 1611–1616.

Boll, F. (1877). Zur Anatomie und Physiologie der Retina. Monatsberichte der Königlich Preussischen Akademie der Wissenschaften zu Berlin, Akademie der Wissenschaften, Berlin: Der KGL, pp. 783–788.

Boll, F. (1878). Zur Physiologie des Sehens und der Farbenempfindung. Monatsberichte der Königlich Preussischen Akademie der Wissenschaften zu Berlin, Akademie der Wissenschaften, Berlin: Der KGL, pp. 2–7.

Boring, E.G. (1957). *A History of Experimental Psychology*. New York: Appleton-Century-Crofts.

Brown, P.K. & Wald, G. (1964). Visual pigments in single rods and cones of the human retina. *Science*, **144**, 45–52.

Buck, S.L. (1985). Cone-rod interaction over time and space. *Vision Research*, **25**, 907–916.

Buck, S.L. (1997). Influence of rod signals on hue perception: evidence from successive contrast. *Vision Research*, **37**, 1295–1301.

Buck, S.L. (2001). What is the hue of rod vision? *Color Research and Application*, **26** (suppl.), S57-S59.

Buck, S.L. (2004). Rod-cone interactions in human vision. In *The Visual Neurosciences*. L.M. Chalupa & J.S. Werner, eds. Cambridge, MA: The MIT Press, pp. 863–878.

Buck, S.L., Knight, R. & Bechtold, J. (2000). Opponent-color models and the influence of rod signals on the loci of unique hues. *Vision Research*, **40**, 3333–3344.

Buck, S.L., Knight, R., Fowler, G. & Hunt, B. (1998). Rod influence on hue-scaling functions. *Vision Research*, **38**, 3259–3263.

Buck, S.L., Peeples, D.R. & Makous, W. (1979). Spatial patterns of rod-cone interaction. *Vision Research*, **19**, 775–782.

Buck, S.L. & Makous, W. (1981). Rod-cone interaction on large and small backgrounds. *Vision Research*, **21**, 1181–1187.

Buck, S.L., Stefurak, D.L., Moss, C. & Regal, D. (1984). The time-course of rod-cone interaction. *Vision Research*, **24**, 543–548.

Burns, M.E. & Lamb, T. (2004). Visual transduction by rod and cone photoreceptors. In *The Visual Neurosciences*. L.M. Chalupa & J.S. Werner, eds. Cambridge, MA: The MIT Press, pp. 215–233.

Cajal, S.R. y (1894). Die Retina der Wirbelthiere. Untersuchungen mit der Golgi-Cajal`schen Chromsil-bermethode und der Ehrlich`schen Methylenblaufärbung. Wiesbaden: Von J.F. Bergmann.

Cajal, S.R. y (1937). *Recollections of My Life. In Memories of the American Philosophical Society, Vol. VIII, Part II, 1937*. Translated by E. Horne Craigie with the assistance of Juan Cano. Philadelphia: The American Philosophical Society.

Cameron, A.M., Mahroo, O.A.R. & Lamb, T.D. (2006). Dark adaptation of human rod bipolar cells measured from the b-wave of the scotopic electroretinogram. *Journal of Physiology*, **575**, 507–526.

Campbell, F.W. & Rushton, W.A.H. (1955). Measurement of the scotopic pigment in the living human eye. *Journal of Physiology*, **130**, 131–147.

Chalmers, A.F. (1986). *What is This Thing Called Science?* Philadelphia: Open University Press.

Cohen, B. (1978). *Isaac Newton's Papers and Letters on Natural Philosophy*. Cambridge, MA: Harvard University Press.

Cone, R.A. (1963/1964). The rat electroretinogram I: contrasting effects of adaptation on the amplitude and latency of the b-wave. *Journal of General Physiology*, **47**, 1089–1105.

Craik, K.J.W. & Vernon, M.D. (1941). The nature of dark adaptation. *British Journal of Psychology*, **32**, 62–81.

Crawford, B.H. (1940). The effect of field size and pattern on the change of visual sensitivity with time. *Proceedings of the Royal Society of London*, B, **129**, 94–106.

Crawford, C.B. (1947). Visual adaptation in relation to brief conditioning stimuli. *Proceedings of the Royal Society of London*, B, **134**, 283–302.

Crozier, W.J. & Wolf, E. (1938/1939). The flicker response contour for the gecko (rod retina). *Journal of General Physiology*, **22**, 555–566.

Daw, N.W., Jensen, R.J. & Brunken, W.J. (1990). Rod pathways in mammalian retinae. *Trends in Neurosciences*, **13**, 110–115.

Dean, D.M., Nguitragool, W., Miri, A., McCabe, S.L. & Zimmerman, A.L. (2002). All-trans-retinal shuts down rod cyclic nucleotide gated ion channels: a novel role for photoreceptor retinoids in response to bright light? *Proceedings of the National Academy of Sciences of the United States of America*, **99** (12), 8372–8377.

De Valois, R.L. (1965). Analysis and coding of color vision in the primate visual system. *Cold Spring Harbor Symposia on Quantitative Biology*, **30**, 567–579.

De Valois, R.L., Abramov, I. & Jacobs, G.H. (1966). Analysis of response patterns of LGN cells. *Journal of the Optical Society of America*, **56**, 966–977.

De Vries, H. (1943). The quantum character of light and its bearing upon threshold of vision, the differential sensitivity and visual acuity of the eye. *Physica*, **10**, 553–564.

Donner, K.O. & Reuter, T. (1968). Visual adaptation of the rhodopsin rods in the frog's retina. *Journal of Physiology*, **199**, 59–87.

Dowling, J.E. (1960). Chemistry of visual adaptation in the rat. *Nature*, **188**, 114–118.

Dowling, J.E. (1967). The site of visual adaptation. *Science*, **155**, 273–279.

Dowling, J.E. & Ripps, H. (1970). Visual adaptation in the retina of the skate. *Journal of General Physiology*, **56**, 491–520.

Dreher, E. (1912). Methodische Untersuchung der Farbentonänderungen homogener Lichter bei zunehmend indirektem Sehen und veränderter Intensität. *Zeitschrift für Sinnesphysiologie*, **46**, 1–82.

Du Croz, J.J. & Rushton, W.A.H. (1966). The separation of cone mechanisms in dark adaptation. *Journal of Physiology*, **183**, 481–496.

Dunn, F.A. & Rieke, F. (2006). The impact of photoreceptor noise on retinal gain controls. *Current Opinion in Neurobiology*, **16**, 363–370.

Ebbinghaus, H. (1893). Theorie des Farbensehens. *Zeitschrift für Psychologie und Physiologie der Sinnesorgane*, **5**, 145–238.

Fain, G.L., Lamb, T.D., Matthews, H.R. & Murphy, R.L.W. (1989). Cytoplasmic calcium as the messenger for light adaptation in salamander rods. *Journal of Physiology*, **416**, 215–243.

Fain, G.L. & Matthews, H.R. (1990). Calcium and the mechanism of light adaptation in vertebrate photoreceptors. *Trends in Neuroscience*, **13**, 378–384.

Fesenko, E.E., Kolosnikov, S.S. & Lyubarsky, A.L. (1985). Induction by cyclic GMP of cationic conductance in plasma membrane of retinal rod outer segment. *Nature*, **313**, 310–313.

Flamant, F. & Stiles, W.S. (1948). The directional and spectral sensitivities of the retinal rods to adapting fields of different wave-lengths. *Journal of Physiology*, **107**, 187–202.

Frumkes, T.E., Sekuler, M.D., Barris, M.C., Reiss, E.H. & Chalupa, L.M. (1973). Rod-cone interaction in human scotopic vision – I. temporal analysis. *Vision Research*, **13**, 1269–1282.

Frumkes, T.E., Sekuler, M.D. & Reiss, E.H. (1972). Rod-cone interaction in human scotopic vision. *Science*, **175**, 913–914.

Frumkes, T.E. & Temme, L.A. (1977). Rod-cone interaction in human scotopic vision: II. Cones influence rod increment thresholds. *Vision Research*, **17**, 673–679.

Goethe, J. W. (1810). Johann Wolfgang Goethe Sämtliche Werke. Briefe, Tagebücher und Gespräche, Band 23/1, In *Johann Wolfgang Goethe zur Farbenlehre*. Manfred Wenzel, ed. (1991). Frankfurt am Main: Deutscher Klassiker Verlag.

Gouras, P. & Link, K. (1966). Rod and cone interaction in dark adapted monkey ganglion cells. *Journal of Physiology*, **184**, 499–510.

Graham, C.H. & Hartline, H.K. (1935). The response of single visual sense cells to lights of different wave-lengths. *Journal of General Physiology*, **18**, 917–931.

Granit, R. (1938). Processes of adaptation in the vertebrate retina in the light of recent photochemical and electrophysiological research. *Documenta Ophthalmologica*, **1**, 7–77.

Granit, R. (1947). *Sensory Mechanisms of the Retina*. London: Oxford University Press.

Granit, R. (1955). *Receptors and Sensory Perception*. New Haven: Yale University Press.

Granit, R. (1963). *Sensory Mechanisms of the Retina, with an Appendix on Electro-retinography*. London: Hafner Publishing Company.

Granit, R., Holmberg, T. & Zewi, M. (1938). On the mode of action of visual purple on the rod cell. *Journal of Physiology*, **94**, 430–440.

Granit, R., Munsterhjelm, A. & Zewi, M. (1939). The relation between concentration of visual purple and retinal sensitivity to light during dark-adaptation. *Journal of Physiology*, **96**, 31–44.

Grassmann, H. von (1853). *Zur Theorie der Farbenmischung. Annalen der Physik und Chemie*. J. C. Poggendorff, ed. Leipzig: von Johann Ambrosius Barth, pp. 69–84.

Greene, B. (2005). *The Fabric of the Cosmos*. London: Penguin Books.

Gribbin, J. (2003). *Science: A History*. London: Penguin Books.

Grünert, U. & Wässle, H. (1996). Glycine receptors in the rod pathway of the macaque monkey retina. *Visual Neuroscience*, **13**, 101–115.

Hanssen, H. S. (2000). *Theofrast fra Eressos*. Kristiansand, Norway: Nordic Academic Press.

Hartline, H.K. (1940). The nerve messages in the fibers of the visual pathway. *Journal of the Optical Society of America*, **30**, 239–247.

Hecht, S. (1919/1920a). The photochemical nature of the photosensory process. *Journal of General Physiology*, **2**, 229–246.

Hecht, S. (1919/1920b). Intensity and the process of photoreception. *Journal of General Physiology*, **2**, 337–347.

Hecht, S. (1919/1920c). The dark adaptation of the human eye. *Journal of General Physiology*, **2**, 499–517.

Hecht, S. (1921/1922). The nature of foveal dark adaptation. *Journal of General Physiology*, **4**, 113–139.

Hecht, S. (1937). Rods, cones, and the chemical basis of vision. *Physiological Review*, **17**, 239–290.

Hecht, S., Haig, C. & Chase, A. (1936/1937). The influence of light adaptation on subsequent dark adaptation of the eye. *Journal of General Physiology*, **20**, 831–850.

Hecht, S., Haig, C. & Wald, G. (1935/1936). The dark adaptation of retinal fields of different size and location. *Journal of General Physiology*, **19**, 321–337.

Hecht, S. & Schlaer, S. (1938). An adaptometer for measuring human dark adaptation. *Journal of the Optical Society of America*, **28**, 269–275.

Helmholtz, H. von (1852). Ueber die Theorie der zusammengesetzten Farben. Annalen der Physik und Chemie, 87 Band, Herausgegeben zu Berlin von J. C. Poggendorff, Johann Ambrosius Barth, Leipzig, pp. 45–66.

Helmholtz, H. von (1855). Ueber die Zusammensetzung von Spektralfarben. Annalen der Physik und Chemie, 94 Band, Herausgegeben zu Berlin von J. C. Poggendorff, Johann Ambrosius Barth, Leipzig, pp. 1–28.

Helmholtz, H. von (1867). *Handbuch der Physiologischen Optik*. Leipzig: Voss.

Helmholtz, H. von (1896). *Handbuch der Physiologischen Optik*. Leipzig: Voss.

Helmholtz, H. von (1911). In *Helmholtz's Treatise on Physiological Optics*. Translated from the third German edition, 1962, James P. C. Southall, ed. New York: Dover Publications, Volumes I and II.

Hering, E. (1878). *Zur Lehre vom Lichtsinne*. Wien: Carl Gerold Sohn`s.

Hering, E. (1964). *Outlines of a Theory of the Light Sense by Evald Hering*. Translated by L. M. Hurvich and D. Jameson. Cambridge, MA: Harvard University Press.

Ingling, C. R. Jr., Lewis, A. L., Loose, D. R. & Myers, K. J. (1977). Cones change rod sensitivity. *Vision Research*, **17**, 555–563.

Kaupp, U. B., Hanke, W., Simmoteit, R. & Lühring, H. (1988). Electrical and biochemical properties of the cGMP-gated cation channel from rod photo- receptors. *Cold Spring Harbor Symposia on Quantitative Biology*, **53**, 407–415.

Kaupp, U. B., Niidome, T., Tanabe, T. *et al.* (1989). Primary structure and functional expression from complementary DNA of the rod photo-receptor cyclic GMP-gated channel. *Nature*, **342**, 762–766.

Kawamura, S. (1993). Rhodopsin phosphorylation as a mechanism of cyclic GMP phosphodiesterase regulation by S-modulin. *Nature*, **362**, 855–857.

Knight, R. & Buck, S. L. (2001). Rod influence on hue perception: effect of background light level. *Color Research and Application*, **26** (suppl.), S60-S64.

Knight, R. & Buck, S. L. (2002). Time-dependent changes of rod influence on hue perception. *Vision Research*, **42**, 1651–1662.

Kohlrausch, A. (1931). Tagessehen, Dämmersehen, Adaptation. In *Handbuch der Normalen und Pathologischen Physiologie*. A. Bethe, G. Bergmann, G. Embden & A. Ellinger, eds. Berlin: Springer, 12 (2), pp. 1499–1594.

König, A. (1894). Über den menschlichen Sehpurpur und seine Bedeutung für das Sehen. Sitzungsberichte der Königlich Preussischen Akademie der Wissenschaften zu Berlin, Zweiter halbband, Juni bis December. Berlin: Der Königlichen Akademie der Wissenschaften, pp. 577–598.

König, A. & Dieterici, C. (1893). Die Grundempfindungen in normalen und anomalen Farbensystemen und ihre Intensitätsverteilung im Spektrum. *Zeitschrift für Psychologie und Physiologie der Sinnesorgane*, **4**, 241–347.

Kries, J. von (1894). Ueber den Einfluss der Adaptation auf Licht- und Farbenempfindung und über die Funktion der Stäbchen. *Berichte der Naturforschenden Gesellschaft zu Freiburg I. B*, **9**, 61–70.

Kries, J. von (1896). Über die Funktion der Netzhautstäbchen. *Zeitschrift für Psychologie und Physiologie der Sinnesorgane*, **9**, 81–123.

Kries, J. von (1911). II. Theories of vision. In *Helmholtz's Treatise on Physiological Optics*. Translated from the third German edition, 1962. J. P. C. Southall, ed. Volumes I and II. New York: Dover Publications, pp. 426–454.

Kries, J. von (1929). Zur Theorie des Tages- und Dämmerungssehens. In *Handbuch der Normalen und Pathologischen Physiologie, Band 12*. A. Bethe, G. Bergmann, G. Embden & A. Ellinger, eds. Berlin: Springer, pp. 679–713.

Kries, J. von & Nagel, W. (1896). Über den Einfluss von Lichtstärke und Adaptation auf das Sehen des Dichromaten (Grünblinden). *Zeitschrift für Psychologie und Physiologie der Sinnesorgane*, **12**, 1–38.

Kuhn, T. S. (1970). *The Structure of Scientific Revolutions*. Chicago: The University of Chicago Press.

Kuhn, T. S. (1994). Reflections on my critics. In *Criticism and the Growth of Knowledge*. Imre Lakatos & Alan Musgrave, eds. Cambridge: Cambridge University Press, pp. 231–278.

Kuffler, S. W. (1953). Discharge patterns and functional organization of mammalian retina. *Journal of Neurophysiology*, **16**, 37–68.

Kühne, W. (1877a). Ueber den Sehpurpur. Untersuchungen aus dem Physiologischen Institute der Universität Heidelberg, Band I, Heft I. Heidelberg: Carl Winter, pp. 15–103.

Kühne, W. (1877b). Ueber die Verbreitung des Sehpurpurs im menschlichen Auge. Untersuchungen aus dem Physiologischen Institute der Universität Heidelberg, Band I, Heft II. Heidelberg: Carl Winter, pp. 105–113.

Kühne, W. (1877–1878). Ueber den Sehpurpur. Untersuchungen aus dem Physiologischen Institute der Universität Heidelberg, Band I & II. Heidelberg: Carl Winter.

Kühne, W. (1879). Chemische Vorgänge in der Netzhaut. *Handbuch der Physiologie*, Dritter Band. Leipzig: Vogel, pp. 235–342.

Lamb, T. D. (1981). The involvement of rod photoreceptors in dark adaptation. *Vision Research*, **21**, 1773–1782.

Lamb, T. D. (1990). Dark adaptation: a re-examination. In *Night Vision, Basic, Clinical and Applied Aspects*. R. F. Hess, L. T. Sharpe & K. Nordby, eds. Cambridge: Cambridge University Press, pp. 177–222.

Latch, M. & Lennie, P. (1977). Rod-cone interaction in light adaptation. *Journal of Physiology*, **269**, 517–534.

Lennie, P. & Fairchild, M. D. (1994). Ganglion cell pathways for rod vision. *Vision Research*, **34**, 477–482.

Lie, I. (1963). Dark adaptation and the photochromatic interval. *Documenta Ophthalmologica*, **17**, 411–510.

Lipetz, L. E. (1961). A mechanism of light adaptation. *Science*, **133**, 639–640.

Loeser, L. (1904). Über den Einfluss der Dunkeladaptation auf die spezifische Farbenschwelle. *Zeitschrift für Psychologie und Physiologie der Sinnesorgane*, **36**, 1–18.

Lythgoe, R. J. (1940). The mechanism of dark adaptation: a critical resumé. *British Journal of Ophthalmology*, **24**, 21–43.

Mach, E. (1865). Über die Wirkung der räumlichen Vertheilung des Lichtreizes auf die Netzhaut. *Sitzungsberichte der Mathematisch-Naturwissenschaftlichen Klasse der Kaiserlichen Akademie der Wissenschaften*, **52**, Abteilung 2, 303–322.

Makous, W. & Booth, R. (1974). Cones block signals from rods. *Vision Research*, **14**, 2285–2294.

Marks, W. B., Dobelle, W. H. & MacNichol, E. F. (1964). Visual pigments of single primate cones. *Science*, **143**, 1181–1182.

Matthews, H. R., Murphy, R. L. W., Fain, G. L. & Lamb, T. D. (1988). Photoreceptor light adaptation is mediated by cytoplasmic calcium concentration. *Nature*, **334**, 67–69.

Maxwell, J. C. (1855). Experiments on colour, as perceived by the eye, with remarks on colour-blindness. From the Transactions of the Royal Society of Edinburgh, Vol. 21; reprinted in *The Scientific Papers of James Clerk Maxwell, 1890*. W. D. Niven, ed. Cambridge: Cambridge University Press, Vol. I, pp. 126–154.

Maxwell, J. C. (1860). On the theory of compound colours, and the relations of the colours of the spectrum. *Philosophical Transactions of the Royal Society of London*, **150**, 57–84.

Maxwell, J. C. (1872). On colour vision. From the Proceedings of the Royal Institution of Great Britain, Vol. 6, 1872; reprinted in *The Scientific Papers of James Clerk Maxwell, 1890*. W. D. Niven, ed. Cambridge: Cambridge University Press, Vol. II, pp. 267–279.

McCabe, S.L., Pelosi, D.M., Tetreault, M. *et al.* (2004). All-trans-retinal is a closed-state inhibitor of rod cyclic nucleotide-gated ion channels. *Journal of General Physiology*, **123**, 521–531.

McCann, J.J. & Benton, J.L. (1969). Interaction of the long-wave cones and the rods to produce colour sensations. *Journal of the Optical Society of America*, **59**, 103–107.

McKee, S.P., McCann, J.J. & Benton, J.L. (1977). Color vision from rod and long-wave cone interactions: conditions in which rods contribute to multicoloured images. *Vision Research*, **17**, 175–185.

Mitarai, G., Svaetichin, G., Vallecalle, E. *et al.* (1961). Glia-neuron interaction and adaptation mechanisms of the retina. In *Neurophysiologie und Psychophysik des visuellen Systems*. R. Jung and H. Kornhuber, eds. Berlin: Springer, pp. 463–481.

Mollon, J.D. & Polden, P.G. (1979). Post-receptoral adaptation. *Vision Research*, **19**, 435–440.

Monod, J. (1970). *Le Hasard et la Nécessité*. Paris: Du Seuil.

Monod, J., Wyman, J. & Changeux, J-P. (1965). On the nature of allosteric transitions: a plausible model. *Journal of Molecular Biology*, **12**, 88–118.

Müller, G.E. (1896). Zur Psychophysik der Gesichtsempfindungen. *Zeitschrift für Psychologie und Physiologie der Sinnesorgane*, Zehnter Band, 321–413.

Müller, G.E. (1897). Zur Psychophysik der Gesichtsempfindungen. Die besondere Funktionsweise der Stäbchen. *Zeitschrift für Psychologie und Physiologie der Sinnesorgane*, Vierzhnter Band, 161–193.

Müller, G.E. (1923). Zur Theorie des Stäbchenapparates und der Zapfenblindheit. Zeitschrift für Psychologie und Physiologie der Sinnesorgane. II. *Abteilung. Zeitschrift für Sinnesphysiologie*, **54** Band, 9–48 and 102–145.

Müller, G.E. (1930). Über die Farbenempfindungen. Zeitschrift für Psychologie und Physiologie der Sinnesorgane. *Ergänzungsband*, **17**, 1–434.

Müller, J. (1840). *Handbuch der Physiologie des Menschen*, Zweiter Band. Coblenz: Verlag von J. Hölscher.

Nagel, W. (1911). Adaptation, twilight vision, and the duplicity theory. In *Handbuch der Physiologischen Optik von H. von Helmholtz* (Dritte Auflage). A. Gullstrand, J. von Kries & W. Nagel, eds. Zweiter Band, Hamburg and Leipzig: Leopold Voss, pp. 313–394.

Naka, K.I. & Rushton, W.H.A. (1968). S-potential and dark adaptation in fish. *Journal of Physiology*, London, **194**, 259–269.

Nerger, J.L., Volbrecht, V.J. & Ayde, C.J. (1995). Unique hue judgments as a function of test size in the fovea and at 20-deg temporal eccentricity. *Journal of the Optical Society of America A*, **12**, 1225–1232.

Nerger, J.L., Volbrecht, V.J., Ayde, C.J. & Imhoff, S.M. (1998). Effect of the S-cone mosaic and rods on red/green equilibria. *Journal of the Optical Society of America A*, **15**, 2816–2826.

Newton, I. (1671/1672). In *Philosophical Transactions of the Royal Society of London*, Vol. 6, 3075–3087.

Newton, I. (1675). In *Isaac Newton's Papers and Letters on Natural Philosophy*. (B. Cohen, ed., second edition, 1978, Cambridge, MA: Harvard University Press, pp. 177–235.)

Newton, I. (1730). *Opticks or a Treatise of the Reflections, Refractions, Inflections and Colours of Light* (based on the fourth edition, London, 1730), Bernard Cohen, ed., 1979. New York: Dover Publications.

Nicol, G.D. & Bownds, M.D. (1989). Calcium regulates some, but not all aspects of light adaptation in rod photoreceptors. *Journal of General Physiology*, **94**, 233–259.

Nordby, K., Stabell, B. & Stabell, U. (1984). Dark-adaptation of the human rod system. *Vision Research*, **24**, 841–849.

Parinaud, H. (1881). L'hemeralopie et les fonctions du pourpre visuel. *Comptes Rendus Hebdomadaires Des Séances De l'Académie des Sciences*, **93**, 286–287.

Parinaud, H. (1884a). Sur la sensibilité visuelle. *Comptes Rendus Hebdomadaires Des Séances De l'Académie des Sciences*, **99**, 241–242.

Parinaud, H. (1884b). De l'intensité lumineuse des couleurs spectrales; influence de l'adaptation rétinienne. *Comptes Rendus Hebdomadaires Des Séances De l'Académie des Sciences*, **99**, 937–939.

Parinaud, H. (1885). Sur l'existence de deux espèces de sensibilité à la lumière. *Comptes Rendus Hebdomadaires Des Séances De l'Académie des Sciences*, **101**, 821–823.

Pepe, I.M., Panfoli, I. & Hamm, H.E. (1989). Visual transduction in vertebrate photoreceptors. *Cell Biophysics*, **14**, 129–137.

Pepperberg, D.R. (1984). Rhodopsin and visual adaptation: photoreceptor thresholds in the isolated skate retina. *Vision Research*, **24**, 357–366.

Perutz, M.F. (1989). Mechanisms of cooperativity and allosteric regulation in proteins. *Quarterly Reviews of Biophysics*, **22** (2), 139–237.

Polden, P.G. & Mollon, J.D. (1980). Reversed effect of adapting stimuli on visual sensitivity. *Proceedings of the Royal Society of London*, B, **210**, 235–272.

Polyak, S.L. (1941/1948). *The Retina*. Chicago: University of Chicago Press.

Popper, K.R. (1969). *Conjectures and Refutations*. London: Routledge & Kegan Paul.

Popper, K.R. (1975). *The Logic of Scientific Discovery*. London: Hutchinson.

Popper, K.R. (1994). Normal science and its dangers. In *Criticism and the Growth of Knowledge*. Imre Lakatos & Alan Musgrave, eds. Cambridge: Cambridge University Press, pp. 51–58.

Pugh, E.N. (1975). Rushton's paradox: rod dark adaptation after flash photolysis. *Journal of Physiology*, **248**, 413–431.

Purkinje, J. (1825). Beobachtungen und Versuche zur Physiologie der Sinne. Neue Beiträge zur Kenntniss des Sehens in subjectiver Hinsicht, Zweiter band. Berlin: Reimer.

Rose, A. (1953). Quantum and noise limitations of the visual process. *Journal of the Optical Society of America*, **43**, 715–716.

Rushton, W.A.H. (1957). Physical measurement of cone pigment in the living human eye. *Nature*, **179**, 571–573.

Rushton, W.A.H. (1961a). Dark-adaptation and the regeneration of rhodopsin. *Journal of Physiology*, **156**, 166–178.

Rushton, W.A.H. (1961b). Rhodopsin measurements and dark-adaptation in a subject deficient in cone vision. *Journal of Physiology*, **156**, 193–205.

Rushton, W.A.H. (1965a). The Ferrier Lecture: visual adaptation. *Proceedings of the Royal Society of London*, B, **162**, 20–46.

Rushton, W.A.H. (1965b). Bleached rhodopsin and visual adaptation. *Journal of Physiology*, **181**, 645–655.

Rushton, W.A.H. (1966). Densitometry of pigments in rods and cones of normal and color defective subjects. *Investigative Ophthalmology*, **5**, 233–241.

Rushton, W.A.H. (1972). Light and dark adaptation. *Investigative Ophthalmology*, **11**, 503–517.

Rushton, W.A.H. & Campbell, F.W. (1954). Measurement of rhodopsin in the living human eye. *Nature*, **174**, 1096–1097.

Rushton, W.A.H., Campbell, F.W., Hagins, W.A. & Brindley, G.S. (1955). The bleaching and regeneration of rhodopsin in the living eye of the albino rabbit and of man. *Optica Acta*, **1**, 183–190.

Rushton, W.A.H., Fulton, A.B. & Baker, H.D. (1969). Dark-adaptation and the rate of pigment regeneration. *Vision Research*, **9**, 1473–1479.

Rushton, W.A.H. & Powell, D.S. (1972a). The early phase of dark adaptation. *Vision Research*, **12**, 1083–1093.

Rushton, W.A.H. & Powell, D.S. (1972b). The rhodopsin content and the visual threshold of human rods. *Vision Research*, **12**, 1073–1081.

Rushton, W.A.H. & Westheimer, G. (1962). The effect upon the rod threshold of bleaching neighbouring rods. *Journal of Physiology*, **164**, 318–329.

Saugstad, P. & Saugstad, A. (1959). The Duplicity Theory: an evaluation. *Advances in Ophthalmology*, **9**, 1–51.

Schjelderup, H.K. (1920). Zur Theorie der Farbenempfindungen. Zeitschrift für Psychologie und Physiologie der Sinnesorgane. II. *Abteilung. Zeitschrift für Sinnesphysiologie*, **51** Band, 19–45.

Schneeweis, D.M. & Schnapf, J.L. (1995). Photovoltage of rods and cones in the macaque retina. *Science*, **268**, 1053–1056.

Schultze, M. (1866). Zur Anatomie und Physiologie der Retina. *Archiv für mikroskopische Anatomie*, Band **2**, 175–286..

Sharpe, L.T. (1990). The light-adaptation of the human rod visual system. In *Night Vision: Basic, Clinical and Applied Aspects*. R.F. Hess, L.T. Sharpe & K. Nordby, eds. Cambridge: Cambridge University Press, pp. 49–124.

Shlaer, S., Smith, E. L. & Chase, A. M. (1941/1942). Visual acuity and illumination in different spectral regions. *Journal of General Physiology*, **25**, 553–569.

Stabell, B. (1967a). Rods as color receptors in scotopic vision. *Scandinavian Journal of Psychology*, **8**, 132–138.

Stabell, B., Nordby, K. & Stabell, U. (1987). Light-adaptation of the human rod system. *Clinical Vision Sciences*, **2**, 83–91.

Stabell, B. & Stabell, U. (1971a). Facilitation of chromatic cone activity by rod activity. I. Red-related cone activity. *Scandinavian Journal of Psychology*, **12**, 99–105.

Stabell, B. & Stabell, U. (1973a). Chromatic rod vision IX: a theoretical survey. *Vision Research*, **13**, 449–450.

Stabell, B. & Stabell, U. (1974). Chromatic rod-cone interaction. *Vision Research*, **14**, 1389–1392.

Stabell, B. & Stabell, U. (1976). Effects of rod activity on color threshold. *Vision Research*, **16**, 1105–1110.

Stabell, B., Stabell, U. & Nordby, K. (1986b). Dark-adaptation in a rod monochromat: effect of stimulus size, exposure time and retinal eccentricity. *Clinical Vision Sciences*, **1**, 75–80.

Stabell, B. & Stabell, U. (1998). Chromatic rod-cone interaction during dark adaptation. *Journal of the Optical Society of America A*, **15**, 2809–2815.

Stabell, U. (1967b). Rods as color receptors in photopic vision. *Scandinavian Journal of Psychology*, **8**, 139–144.

Stabell, U. & Stabell, B. (1965). Rods as color receptors. *Scandinavian Journal of Psychology*, **6**, 195–200.

Stabell, U. & Stabell, B. (1971b). Facilitation of chromatic cone activity by rod activity. II. Variation of chromatic-related cone activity. *Scandinavian Journal of Psychology*, **12**, 168–174.

Stabell, U. & Stabell, B. (1971c). Chromatic rod vision II: wavelength of pre-stimulation varied. *Scandinavian Journal of Psychology*, **12**, 282–288.

Stabell, U. & Stabell, B. (1973b). Chromatic rod activity at mesopic intensities. *Vision Research*, **13**, 2255–2260.

Stabell, U. & Stabell, B. (1975). Scotopic contrast hues triggered by rod activity. *Vision Research*, **15**, 1115–1118.

Stabell, U. & Stabell, B. (1978). Scotopic hues of simultaneous contrast. *Vision Research*, **18**, 1491–1496.

Stabell, U. & Stabell, B. (1989). Dark-adaptation mechanisms of the long-wave cones. *Scandinavian Journal of Psychology*, **30**, 207–219.

Stabell, U. & Stabell, B. (1994). Mechanisms of chromatic rod vision in scotopic illumination. *Vision Research*, **34**, 1019–1027.

Stabell, U. & Stabell, B. (1996). Long-term rod dark adaptation in man: threshold measurements, rhodopsin regeneration and allosteric sensitivity regulation. An evaluation. *Scandinavian Journal of Psychology*, **37**, 259–268.

Stabell, U., Stabell, B. & Fugelli, A. (1992). Mechanisms of long-term dark adaptation. *Scandinavian Journal of Psychology*, **33**, 12–19.

Stabell, U., Stabell, B., Hisdal, B. & Nordby, K. (1990). Rod and cone dark adaptation. *Clinical Vision Sciences*, **4**, 345–351.

Stabell, U., Stabell, B. & Nordby, K. (1986a). Dark-adaptation of the human rod system: a new hypothesis. *Scandinavian Journal of Psychology*, **27**, 175–183.

Stabell, U., Stabell, B. & Nordby, K. (1989). On the photochemical theory of dark adaptation. In *Basic Issues in Psychology*. I.A. Bjørgen, ed. London: Sigma, pp. 247–254.

Stiles, W.S. (1939). The directional sensitivity of the retina and the spectral sensitivities of the rods and cones. *Proceedings of the Royal Society of London*, B, **127**, 64–105.

Stiles, W.S. (1978). *Mechanisms of Colour Vision: Selected Papers of W.S. Stiles F.R. S. with a New Introductory Essay*. London: Academic Press.

Stiles, W.S. & Crawford, B.A. (1932). Equivalent adaptation levels in localized retinal areas. Report of a joint discussion on vision held on 3 June 1932 at the Imperial College of Science by the Physical and Optical Societies. London: Cambridge University Press.

Stromeyer III, C.F. (1974a). Form-specific colour after effects in scotopic illumination. *Nature*, **250**, 266–268.

Stromeyer III, C.F. (1974b). Rod signals in higher color mechanisms: the McCollough color aftereffect observed in scotopic illumination. In *Sensation and Measurement*. H.R. Moskowitz, B. Scharf & J.C. Stevens, eds. Boston: Reidel, pp. 403–410.

Svaetichin, G. (1953). The cone action potential. *Acta Physiologica Scandinavica*, **106**, 565–600.

Tansley, K. (1931). The regeneration of visual purple: its relation to dark adaptation and night blindness. *Journal of Physiology*, **71**, 442–458.

Temme, L.A. & Frumkes, T.E. (1977). Rod-cone interaction in human scotopic vision III: rods influence cone increment thresholds. *Vision Research*, **17**, 681–685.

Trezona, P.W. (1960). The after-effects of a white light stimulus. *Journal of Physiology*, **150**, 67–78.

Trezona, P.W. (1970). Rod participation in the 'blue' mechanism and its effect on colour matching. *Vision Research*, **10**, 317–332.

Tschermak, A. (1902). Die Hell-Dunkeladaptation des Auges und die Funktion der Stäbchen und Zapfen. In *Ergebnisse der Physiologie*. L. Asher & K. Spiro, eds. Erster Jahrgang, II. Abteilung, Bergmann: Wiesbaden, Biophysik und Psychophysik, pp. 695–800.

Tschermak, A. (1929). Theorie des Farbensehens. In *Handbuch der Normalen und Pathologischen Physiologie*. A. Bethe, G. Bergmann, G. Embden & A. Ellinger, eds. Band 12 (1), Berlin: Springer, pp. 550–584.

Volbrecht, V.J., Nerger, J.L., Imhoff, S.M. & Ayde, C.J. (2000). Effect of the short-wavelength-sensitive-cone mosaic and rods on the locus of unique green. *Journal of the Optical Society of America A*, **17**, 628–634.

Wald, G. (1933). Vitamin A in the retina. *Nature*, **132**, 316–317.

Wald, G. (1934). Carotenoids and the vitamin A cycle in vision. *Nature*, **134**, 65.

Wald, G. (1934/1935). Vitamin A in eye tissues. *Journal of General Physiology*, **18**, 905–915.

Wald, G. (1935/1936). Carotenoids and the visual cycle. *Journal of General Physiology*, **19**, 351–371.

Wald, G. (1937a). Visual purple system in fresh-water fishes. *Nature*, **139**, 1017–1018.

Wald, G. (1937b). Photo-labile pigments of the chicken retina. *Nature*, **140**, 545–546.

Wald, G. (1937/1938). Area and visual threshold. *Journal of General Physiology*, **21**, 269–287.

Wald, G. (1938/1939). The porphyropsin visual system. *Journal of General Physiology*, **22**, 775–794.

Wald, G. (1949a). The photochemistry of vision. *Documenta Ophthalmologica*, **3**, 94–137.

Wald, G. (1949b). The enzymatic reduction of the retinenes to the vitamin A. *Science*, **109**, 482–483.

Wald, G. (1954). On the mechanism of the visual threshold and visual adaptation. *Science*, **119**, 887–892.

Wald, G. (1958). The Selig Hecht Commemorative Lecture. Retinal chemistry and the physiology of vision. In *Visual Problems of Colour*. London: Her Majesty's Stationery Office, National Physical Laboratory Symposium No. 8, Vol. 1, pp. 7–61.

Wald, G. (1964). The receptors of human color vision. *Science*, **145**, 1007–1017.

Wald, G. (1967). Blue-blindness in the normal fovea. *Journal of the Optical Society of America*, **57**, 1289–1301.

Wald, G. (1968). Molecular basis of visual excitation. *Science*, **162**, 230–239.

Walters, H. V. & Wright, W. D. (1943). The spectral sensitivity of the fovea and extrafovea in the Purkinje range. *Proceedings of the Royal Society of London*, B, **131**, 340–361.

Weale, R. A. (1957). Trichromatic ideas in the seventeenth and eighteenth centuries. *Nature*, **179**, 648–651.

Westheimer, G. (1965). Spatial interaction in the human retina during scotopic vision. *Journal of Physiology*, **181**, 881–894.

Westheimer, G. (1968). Bleached rhodopsin and retinal interaction. *Journal of Physiology*, **195**, 97–105.

Westheimer, G. (1970). Rod-cone independence for sensitizing interaction in the human retina. *Journal of Physiology*, **206**, 109–116.

Wiesel, T. N. & Hubel, D. H. (1966). Spatial and chromatic interactions in the lateral geniculate body of the rhesus monkey. *Journal of Neurophysiology*, **29**, 1115–1156.

Willmer, E. N. (1946). *Retinal Structure and Colour Vision*. Cambridge: Cambridge University Press.

Willmer, E. N. (1950). Low threshold rods and the perception of blue. *Journal of Physiology*, **11**, 17P.

Willmer, E. N. (1961). Human colour vision and the perception of blue. *Journal of Theoretical Biology*, **2**, 141–179.

Wright, W.D. (1946). *Researches on Normal and Defective Colour Vision*. London: Henry Kimpton,.

Wässle, H., Grünert, U., Chun, M-H. & Boycott, B.B. (1995). The rod-pathway of the macaque monkey retina: identification of AII-amacrine cells with antibodies against calretinin. *The Journal of Comparative Neurology*, **361**, 537–551.

Yeh, T., Lee, B.B. & Kremers, J. (1996). The time course of adaptation in macaque retinal ganglion cells. *Vision Research*, **36**, 913–931.

Yin, L., Smith, R.G., Sterling, P. & Brainard, D.H. (2006). Chromatic properties of horizontal and ganglion cell responses follow a dual gradient in cone opsin expression. *Journal of Neuroscience*, **26** (47), 12351–12361.

Young, T. (1802a). The Bakerian Lecture. On the theory of light and colours. *Philosophical Transactions of the Royal Society of London*, **92**, 12–48.

Young, T. (1802b). An account of some cases of the production of colours, not hitherto described. *Philosophical Transactions of the Royal Society of London*, **92**, 387–397.

Young, T. (1807). Lecture 37: on physical optics. *A Course of Lectures on Natural Philosophy and the Mechanical Arts*, Vol. I. London: William Savage Bedford Bury, pp. 434–446.

Index

Printed in the United States
By Bookmasters